"Heart Disease: What Your Doctor Won't Tell You
is a great challenge to the claims and practices
of mainstream medical science. With its publication,
the most responsible profession on earth has been
called to enter a new phase of its history: reformation."

—Ernest Dempsey,
author and reviewer

Many manufacturers and sellers claim trademarks on their unique products. When these trademarks appear in this book and we are aware of them, we have used initial capital letters (e.g., Prozac) for designation.

Endnotes designated in the text of this book can be found at the end of each chapter. Patient testimonials are based on actual experiences as observed by the author. Patient names have been changed to protect privacy.

Printed in the United States of America.
Harrison and Hampton Publishing, Inc.
2700 Rogers Drive, Suite 204
Birmingham AL 35209
1-888-884-9577
(205) 879-2383

Editing and book design by Betsy Stokes
Cover design by Mike McCracken

This book and the advice given are not intended to take the place of your physician. The author recommends that all patients consult with a medical doctor before discontinuing any prescription medication.

This book is distributed by Cardinal Publishers Group
2402 N. Shadeland Ave, suite A
Indianapolis, IN 46219
info@cardinalpub.com
(317) 352-8200

Heart Disease

What Your Doctor Won't Tell You

Dr. Rodger H. Murphree II, DC, CNS

Table of Contents

Introduction

It's been a long day at work, and as you're pulling into your driveway, you begin to have chest pain. The pain stops you cold in your tracks; it takes your breath away. The pressure eases a bit but then starts up again, and pain is now radiating to your left arm and jaw. Your head is spinning. It feels like you have an elephant sitting on your chest. You can't breathe, and you start to feel faint.

Stumbling into the house, you call out for your wife (or husband), who immediately sees that something is wrong. Surely you must be having a heart attack. She calls 9-1-1, and you are rushed to the emergency room where a horde of medical staff descend on you, pump you full of questions while drawing your blood, and hook you to a heart monitor.

Life-saving drugs are administered to open up your arteries, and an immediate angiogram is ordered. The heart surgeon reports that the angiogram demonstrates blockages in the arteries leading to your heart. He recommends bypass surgery right away: "I can't be responsible if you decide to leave here without having surgery. You're a walking time bomb." You have a tough decision, my friend.

Filled with panic, pain, and the numbing affect of fatigue, you are tempted to agree with whatever the doctor recommends. The surgeon, nurses, hospital staff, and even your spouse are pressuring you to have the surgery. Should you? You may not know that as many as 10% of those who have bypass surgery die from the procedure. Did you know that 53% of those undergoing bypass surgery will have brain damage that will cause mental disturbances (depression, senility, memory loss, etc.) for up to five years after the surgery? Did you know that many of the drugs used to treat heart disease and hypertension actually accelerate heart disease? Nobody mentioned that?

A New Philosophy of Treatment

Sixty-eight million Americans suffer from some form of heart disease. Over one million Americans have a heart attack each year. Nearly one million die each year from cardiovascular related illnesses. That's 41% of all annual deaths in the United States.[1]

In fact, cardiovascular disease claims as many lives as the next eight leading causes of death combined—including cancer, accidents, and AIDS. Let's put it in a more short-term perspective. About one person dies every 33 seconds from heart disease. This is 2,600 deaths a day! And the issue isn't only in the United States. Heart disease is responsible for 50% of all deaths worldwide.[2]

Traditional medicine and its political organizations—including the American Heart Association—have failed to stem the rising tide of heart disease. For all their best intentions, many of our busy, overworked doctors have to simply make do with what they've been taught. They don't have time to test their theories, follow up with their patients, or meditate on their results. We clearly need a new approach. And it must be based on truths, not medical myths.

As if the title isn't clear enough, I'll warn you that this isn't another book filled with recycled, outdated information that simply tows the party line. The material I'm presenting will likely be quite different from any you've seen in regards to heart disease.

Like many things in life, heart disease—also known as coronary artery disease (CAD)—is a complicated matter. Still, there are quite a number of experts who are ready to tell you they have all the answers (even if their answers have been proven wrong). This book was spawned from my desire to help my patients sift through the well-meant but false medical advice associated with heart disease.

As the owner and clinical director of a large integrative medical practice, I treated numerous medical misfits who became medical miracles. These were the patients who had tried everything traditional medicine had to offer, only to be told, "There is nothing more we can do for you." Many at first could barely walk more than a few yards without having chest pain and difficulty breathing. Yet they recovered quite well on our integrative approach, which combines judicious use of prescription drugs, diet changes, chelation therapy, and nutritional supplementation.

Science, Not Propaganda

As you'll soon learn, relying on medical myths to prevent and treat cardiovascular disease is hazardous to your health. Fortunately, there are numerous well-researched, clinically proven therapies that don't rely on dangerous drugs or pseudoscience.

In the first several chapters, I attempt to make plain the results of some respected scientific studies that shake up the traditional medical model for understanding and treating heart disease. If you'll take the time to read this book, you'll know more than many of today's medical doctors and certainly more than 99% of the population. You'll certainly be better prepared to live a long and healthy life free of high blood pressure and complications from mitral valve prolapse, heart disease, or dangerous drugs. Given heart disease's epidemic proportions and that several of the therapies used to treat it actually cause more deaths than they save, you can consider this book a wise investment in your health.

Many of the scientific studies contained in this book are not commonly known. And most conventional medical doctors would be amazed to learn that their views on surgery, drugs, and even the causes of heart disease are being called into question by current scientific research. As you'll soon read, however, results from medical studies published in journals such as the *New England Journal of Medicine,* the *Lancet,* and the *British Medical Journal* strongly suggest that we must change our commonly held views on the causes of heart disease and hypertension—as well as our approach to their treatment.

Notes

1. "Heart Disease and Stroke Statistics," American Heart Association (2008), www.americanheart.org/presenter.jhtml?identifier=7016.
2. "Statistics Related to Heart Disease," The Reading Hospital and Medical Center (2008), www.readinghospital.org/health/content.asp?PageID=p06601.

I

Health Care or Disease Care?

Today's standard, American Medical Association–approved medicine is rooted in treating symptoms rather than causes. Its dependence on drugs and surgery is ruinously expensive to patients, insurance companies, and society as a whole.

—Derrick Lonsdale, MD,
Why I Left Orthodox Medicine[1]

Our current AMA-dominated health-care paradigm is based on controlling symptoms. Conventional medicine has made very little progress in correcting the causes associated with two of today's most devastating illnesses, heart disease and cancer. Billions of dollars are spent on battling the much-maligned cholesterol, even though this approach clearly isn't working and may be the cause of an increase in heart-failure rates. When drugs don't control the symptoms, then invasive surgeries are recommended.

Before you assume that I'm antidrug or antisurgery, please know that this is not the case. I do believe in the appropriate use of drugs and surgery. A few years ago, I chopped my finger off in an accident with a lawn mower…an embarrassing story. I was ever so grateful for the surgeon who masterfully repaired my injury. And I was also thankful for the prescription pain pills. Emergency medical procedures save thousands of lives every year. Antibiotics and other drugs prevent millions from dying from diseases that used to routinely mean a death sentence. Insulin-replacement therapy has helped millions of diabetics live more normal lives. Prescription medications provide relief from a number of miserable symptoms. However, all medications are associated with side effects, and the majority don't cure anything.

> *Most over-the-counter, and almost all prescribed, drug treatments merely mask symptoms.... Drugs almost never deal with the reasons why these problems exist, while they frequently create new health problems as side effects of their activities.*
>
> —John R. Lee, MD[2]

Our Symptom-Driven Culture

We now have a pill for every symptom we can describe: poor sleep, depression, constipation, poor digestion, anxiety, fatigue, headaches, diffuse pain, erectile dysfunction, hair loss, sinusitis, hay fever, and more. And the makers of these pills aren't bashful about saturating the TV, radio, newspapers, and magazines with reasons why you need to be taking them. Drug companies are all too happy to provide us with an abundance of synthetic, potentially dangerous drugs for everything that might ail us.

"Are you having trouble sleeping at night?" the commercial asks. "Why not ask your doctor about taking [the latest pill that is supposed to make you feel like the model on the commercial]?" Each year, Americans consume five billion sleeping pills. And each year, thousands of Americans die from them.

Driven by Money, not Health

Since over $400 billion is spent on prescription drugs worldwide, profits are soaring for drug companies. The top 10 companies reported combined profits of $35.9 billion dollars in 2002. This is more than the remaining 490 Fortune 500 companies put together ($33.7 billion). These same drug companies spent $36 billion on advertising and marketing in 2002.[3] It's no wonder we can't escape all the erectile dysfunction ads on TV. Whether or not the drugs work, the ads sure do!

But drugs have to be expensive, right? All that money for research and development has to come from somewhere. Don't believe it! In reality, in 2002 (the date of an extensive nonprofit investigation), only about 14% of Fortune 500 drug-company revenues were applied toward research and development. Over 30% were devoted toward marketing and administration. Around 17% was received as profit.[4] The Families USA, a nonprofit organization, reports that the former CEO of Bristol-Meyers Squibb made $74,890,918 in 2001. This doesn't include his $76,095,611 of unexercised stock options. The chairman of Wyeth pharmaceuticals made over $40 million dollars, exclusive of an additional $40 million in stock options![5] Remember this when you wonder why your health-insurance premiums continue to rise.

Pharmaceutical companies know that in order to make a profit, they must do one of three things: create new illnesses (such as heartburn, erectile dysfunction, social anxiety disorder, or shyness) for their new drugs to treat; get patients to ask for newer, more expensive drugs; or have doctors write more prescriptions, preferably for more expensive "me-too" drugs.

What are "me-too" drugs? They are newer, more expensive versions of older drugs. Between 1998 and 2002, the FDA approved 415 new drugs. Only 14% of these newly approved drugs were actually uniquely different or innovative in their design. The other 86% were old drug formulas masquerading as new innovative therapies. You see, drug companies hoping for FDA approval are only required to prove that new drugs are safe, not that they are more effective than older drugs.[6]

Dr. Marcia Angell, former editor of The *New England Journal of Medicine,* discusses these "me-too" drugs in her book, *The Truth About the Drug Companies.* Take, for instance, the drug Nexium (perhaps you already do). Its creator, AstraZeneca, had been relying on the drug Prilosec for a significant portion of its yearly profits—$6 billion—in 2000.

However, Prilosec was going to lose its patent in 2001, and the folks at AstraZeneca were probably experiencing some heartburn at the thought. Faced with the potential for significant revenue loss, the company simply took one of the two patentable metabolites (chemicals) out of Prilosec and remarketed it as the new and improved Nexium. This "purple pill" then became the original TV drug, as we can all recall. And even though a one-month supply of Nexium costs almost nine times that of the over-the-counter version of Prilosec ($180 compared to $23), the public and their doctors have happily gone along for the ride. The truth? Studies show that both drugs work equally well at reducing stomach acid.[7]

Also consider clot-dissolving medications, which can be lifesaving if given immediately at the onset of a heart attack. There are three different ones on the market. The most prescribed one (tissue plasminogen activator) costs $3,500 for a single dose; the least prescribed one costs $250. Studies show *no difference* in their effectiveness. It's not quality that's driving these increased prescriptions; it's marketing.

Techniques of Greed

So how do drug companies get doctors to prescribe similarly made yet more costly new drugs? Partly through the assault of marketing giveaways by more than 80,000 drug reps who gave away $11 billion worth of free samples.[8] (This amounts to one drug rep for every doctor in the United States.) Bottom-line results clearly show that free samples, vacation "workshop" retreats to posh resorts, and free "educational" gourmet dinners do in fact sway the opinions of doctors. Even more effective, of course, is cash. It's not unusual for drug companies to pay doctors hundred of thousands of dollars a year in "consulting fees." In 2005, drug companies paid for hundreds of millions of dollars and up to 80% of the costs of all doctors' continuing-education classes.[9] Many doctors are paid handsomely to speak on behalf of the drug companies at conferences held at vacation destinations. Through the promise of increased wealth, the drug companies continue to persuade and even brainwash many conventional medical doctors. And as we've already seen, it works.

> *The result of all those attractive women in short skirts armed with pseudoscience invading the practices of doctors is that Americans are over-medicated, taking far too many drugs, most of which they don't even need, and they are paying too much for them.*
>
> —Jerome Kassirer, MD,
> distinguished professor,
> Tufts University School of Medicine[10]

Of course, drug companies must aggressively court both doctors and patients alike because their drugs don't even work for most people. Dr. Allen Rose, a top executive at GlaxoSmithKline, reports that drugs work for as few as 25% of those who take them.[11,12]

In fact, drug companies spend more money on lobbying than does any other industry. There are now two drug lobbyists for every member of Congress.[13]

> *I'm not that hopeful for any real change.... They have bought politicians and doctors. They've looked at everyone and anyone who could stand in their way and they've thrown money at them. The only hope we have is a grassroots revolution that will make the politicians decide they love votes more than drug company money.*
>
> —Dr. Marcia Angell, MD,
> former editor, *New England Journal of Medicine.*[14]

Melody Peterson, former medical reporter for the *New York Times* and author of *Our Daily Meds,* reports from behind-the-scenes interviews with the leading drug companies of the world:

> *In this profit-driven world of medicine, I did not often hear the executives talk of cures. Instead, they focused like honeybees circling a picnic cake on products for what they called chronic disorders. These were drugs that did not cure but 'managed' disease as patients took them once a day for the rest of their lives.*
>
> —Melody Peterson, *Our Daily Meds*[15]

Not only are drug companies seeking out chronic diseases to "manage," they're creating new diseases to market, too. In 2003, the magazine *Medical Marketing and Media* ran an article by Vince Parry who was happy to report that pharmaceutical companies were taking the "art of branding a condition" to ever higher levels of expertise. The focus on developing new disorders (diseases) was apparently all the buzz in the industry.[16]

Medical Myths are Keeping Us Sick

The American Medical Association, American Heart Association, American Diabetes Association, and other conventional medical organizations continue to promote the medical myth that prescription drugs are safer and more effective than more natural alternatives. Unfortunately, while conventional medical doctors are writing record numbers of prescriptions each year, the health of our nation continues to decline. The Centers for Medicare and Medicaid reports that the nation spent $140.6 billion in the year 2000 on prescription drugs.[17] And of course this number escalates each year. It is estimated that over 3 billion prescriptions were written last year.[18]

But even though the United States spends more money on health care per capita than does any other country in the world, The World Health Organization in 2000 ranked the U.S. health-care system first in both responsiveness and cost, but 37th in overall performance and 72nd in overall health (among 191 member nations included in the study).[19]

Dangerous Drugs

In January 1999, *Business Week* reported on the fourth leading cause of hospitalizations: damage from FDA-approved drugs. This affects 2.2 million people a year at a cost of $5 billion. Americans are dying—one every three to five minutes—from the effects of FDA-approved pharmaceutical drugs…used as directed![20] In fact, iatrogenic (accidentally doctor-induced) illnesses take the lives of over 780,000 Americans each year. [21] This makes conventional medicine the number one cause of death in the United States, beating out heart disease and cancer! (And this number is conservative, since only 5–20% of all iatrogenic events are ever reported.)[22]

It's estimated by some experts that adverse drug reactions affect as many as 5 million Americans each year.[23] This is assuredly a conservative estimate. The average U.S. citizen filled 12 prescriptions in 2006,[24] and over a lifetime of drug taking, he or she has a 26% chance of being hospitalized from a drug injury. Yet these same drugs—taken as directed—kill over 270 Americans *each day.* This is comparable to a commercial jet going down on a daily basis! The very drugs that are being used to treat various illnesses are causing more American deaths in one year than occurred in the entire Vietnam War.[25]

Still, medical drug use continues to increase in the United States. Americans now spend over $250 billion a year on prescription drugs, more than the gross domestic product of most countries in the world. Drugs are now the fastest growing part of the staggeringly high American health-care bill. In fact, Americans spend more on drugs than do all the people in Australia, Canada, France, Germany, Italy, Japan, Spain, Brazil, Argentina, Mexico, New Zealand, and the United Kingdom combined![26]

And many of these prescriptions aren't safe at all. For instance, calcium channel blockers—used to treat high blood pressure and heart disease—actually increase the risk of stroke and heart attack five times, according to Dr. Curt Furberg, Wake Forest School of Medicine.[27] And Propulsid—a drug used to treat GERD (gastroesophageal reflux disease) and gastroparesis (delayed emptying of the stomach, usually found in type-2 diabetics)—has caused severe heart-rhythm abnormalities. In June 1998, the FDA issued a statement reporting 38 deaths in the United States from people taking Propulsid: "Due to reports of serious heart arrhythmias and deaths in people taking Propulsid (Cisapride), the label had been changed to reflect these dangers."[28]

Perhaps more subtle, but certainly serious, are drug-induced nutritional deficiencies.[29] Although these can be corrected early, they often aren't, because conventional medicine tends to gloss over such "minor" concerns. Have you taken any of the drugs on the next page? Did *any*one recommend that you give attention to the nutritional depletions destined to accompany your treatment?

- **Aspirin** depletes folic acid, iron, potassium, sodium, and vitamin C.
- **Beta blockers** deplete coenzyme Q10 (CoQ10), an important nutrient for liver function and for cardiovascular and overall health. This can lead to heart disease, fatigue, and muscle pain.
- **Amitriptyline** (Elavil) depletes CoQ10 and vitamin B2. This can cause headaches, anxiety, depression, heart disease, fatigue, and muscle pain.
- **Carbamazepine** (Tegratol) depletes biotin, folic acid, and vitamin D. This can cause pain, fatigue, and depression.
- **Celecoxib** (Celebrex) depletes folic acid. This can cause anxiety and depression.
- **Corticosteroids** (cortisone, dexamethasone, hydrocortisone, prednisone) deplete calcium, folic acid, magnesium, potassium, selenium, vitamin C, vitamin D, and zinc.This can cause depression, fatigue, pain, heart disease, and other illnesses.
- **Digoxin** (Lanoxin) depletes calcium, magnesium, phosphorus, and vitamin B1.
- **Estrogens** (Estrace, Estratab, Estrostep, Menest, Premarin) deplete magnesium, omega-3 fatty acids, vitamin B6, and zinc. This can cause pain, depression, poor immune function, and other illnesses.
- **Famotidine** (Pepcid and Pepcid AC) depletes calcium, folic acid, iron, vitamin B12, vitamin D, and zinc. This can cause poor immune function, fatigue, depression, and pain.
- **Hydrochlorothiazide** (Esidrix, Ezide, Dyazide, DydroDIURIL, Hydro-Par, Maxide, Microzide, Oretic) depletes CoQ10, magnesium, potassium, vitamin B6, and zinc. This can cause pain, fatigue, depression, restless leg syndrome, irritable bowel syndrome, spastic colon, and other illnesses.
- **Nonsteroidal anti-inflammatory drugs** (fenoprofen, ibuprofen, neproxen, Aleve, Anaprox, Advil, Excedrin, Motrin, Naprosyn, Nuprin, Orudis, Pamprin) deplete folic acid. This can cause anxiety and depression.
- **Omeprazole** (Prilosec) depletes vitamin B12.This can lead to fatigue, anemia, and depression.
- **Oral contraceptives** deplete vitamin C, vitamin B2, folic

acid, magnesium, vitamin B6, vitamin B12, and zinc. This could lead to poor immune function, anxiety, depression, and fatigue.

- **Prevastatin** (Pravachol) depletes CoQ10. This could cause heart disease, fatigue, and muscle pain.
- **Ranitidine hydrochloride** (Zantac) depletes calcium, folic acid, iron, vitamin B12, vitamin D, and zinc. This could cause poor immune function, fatigue, depression, anxiety, restless leg syndrome, anemia, and more.
- **Triamterine** (Dyrenium) depletes calcium, folic acid, and zinc. This could cause fatigue, depression, anxiety, and poor immunity.
- **Valproic acid** (Depacote) depletes carnitine and folic acid. This could contribute to diabetes and cause depression and fatigue.
- **Statin drugs** (Lipitor, Crestor, Zocor) block production of CoQ10. This action can lead to muscle aches and pains.

Conventional Medicine and Heart Disease

Almost without exception, conventional cardiologists will discourage you from looking at less dangerous yet equally effective alternatives to prescription medications and surgery. They are convinced that these are not only the best way, but the only way, to treat heart disease and high blood pressure. However, as we'll see in the next chapter, the conventional medical therapies used to treat heart disease and high blood may cause more harm than good.

NOTES

1. Derrick Lonsdale, *Why I Left Orthodox Medicine* (Charlottesville, VA: Hampton Roads, 1994).
2. John R. Lee and Virginia Hopkins, *What Your Doctor May Not Tell You About Menopause* (New York: Warner, 2004).
3. Public Citizen, "2002 Drug Industry Profits: Hefty Pharmaceutical Company Margins Dwarf Other Industries," Congress Watch (June 2003), www.citizen.org/congress/reform/drug_industry/corporate/articles.cfm?ID=9923.
4. ibid.
5. Families USA, "Profiting from Pain: Where Prescription Drug Dollars Go," Publication 02-105 (July 2002), www.familiesusa.org/assets/pdfs/PPreport89a5.pdf.
6. Marcia Angell, *The Truth About the Drug Companies* (New York: Random House, 2004).
7. ibid.
8. Tyler Chin, "Drug Firms Score by Paying Doctors for Time," *American Medical News* (May 6, 2001).
9. Arnold S. Relman, "Defending Professional Independence: ACCME's Proposed New Guidelines for Commercial Support of CME," *Journal of the American Medical Association* 89 (2003): : 2418–2420.
10. Jerome P. Kassirer, "How Drug Lobbyists Influence Doctors," editorial, *Boston Globe* (February 13, 2006).
11. Spear et al., "Clinical Application of Pharmacogenetics," *Trends in Molecular Medicine* (May 2001).
12. Steve Connor, "Glaxo Chief: Our Drugs Do Not Work on Most People," *The Independent* (December 8, 2003).
13. Public Citizen, "The Other Drug War II: Drug Companies Deploy an Army of 623 Lobbyists to Keep Profits Up," Congress Watch (June 2002), www.citizen.org/congress/reform/drug_industry/contribution/articles.cfm?ID=7908.
14. Jerome P. Kassirer, "How Drug Lobbyists Influence Doctors."
15. Melody Petersen, *Our Daily Meds: How the Pharmaceutical Companies Transformed Themselves into Slick Marketing Machines and Hooked the Nation on Prescription Drugs* (New York: Sarah Crichton, 2008): 19.
16. Vince Parry, "The Art of Branding a Condition," *Medical Marketing and Media* (May 2003).
17. Rachel Christensen Sethl and the Employee Research Institute, "Prescription Drugs: Recent Trends in Utilization," *Expenditures and Coverage* 265 (January 2004).
18. Pennsylvania Health Care Cost Containment Council, "Prescription Drug Safety," PHC4 FYI (May, 2004), www.phc4.org/reports/fyi/fyi25.htm.
19. "World Health Organization Assesses the World's Health System," press release of the World Health Organization (June 21, 2000).
20. Daniel Haley, "The Other Drug War," *Alternative Medicine* 43 (September 2001).

21. Categories included are deaths from adverse drug reactions, medical errors, bedsores, infection, malnutrition, outpatient treatment, unnecessary procedures, and complications related to surgery.
22. Gary Null et al., "Death by Medicine," *Life Extension,* web special (March 2004), www.lef.org/magazine/mag2004/mar2004_awsi_death_01.htm.
23. D.W. Bates, "Drugs and Adverse Reactions: How Worried Should We Be?" *Journal of the American Medical Association* 279(15) (1998): 1216–7.
24. Kaiser Family Foundation, from calculations using data from IMS Health, www.imshealth.com.
25. Gary Null et al., "Death by Medicine," *Life Extension,* web special (March 2004), www.lef.org/magazine/mag2004/mar2004_awsi_death_01.htm.
26. Melody Peterson, *Our Daily Meds: How the Pharmaceutical Companies Transformed Themselves into Slick Marketing Machines and Hooked the Nation on Prescription Drugs* (New York: Sarah Crichton, 2008).
27. Curt Furberg and Bruce Psaty, Epidemiology and Prevention Council of the American Heart Association, meeting notes, San Antonio (March 10, 1995).
28. Letter to doctors from Janssen Pharmacuetica, June 26, 1998, www.fda.gov/medwatch/safety/1998/propul.htm.
29. Carrie Louise Daenell, "Drug Induced Nutrient Deficiencies," www.naturalhealthsolution.com/nutrientdeficiencies.htm.

2

Dangerous Drugs

BEFORE I LAUNCH INTO MY ATTACK on cardiovascular drugs, please understand: I don't make up this stuff; I just report it. Unless otherwise notes, most of the material you are about to read comes right out of the "Monthly Prescribing Guide" of the *Physicians' Desk Reference,*[1] the doctor's bible for prescription drugs. It's the same information you're usually given when you purchase your prescription drug. It's just that I present it in type large enough to actually read.

But I can understand why the type is so small on those prescription inserts. There's a lot of information—and warnings—to include. But we often just gloss right over it all. Due to the never-ending promotion of a drug for every ailment, we've become jaded to the potential side effects of various prescription medications.

And why bother reading, when we can just take the T.V. actors' word for it? They seem so happy and symptom-free while that positive, inflected, mind-numbing voice in the background dictates, "In clinical trials, this drug had the following minor side effects: headaches, diarrhea, nausea, coughing, bladder infections, depression, suicidal thoughts, colitis, fever blisters, weakened immune system, and shyness. Do not take if you ever hope to become pregnant with a healthy child. Tell your doctor if you start to die, as this may be a sign of a serious side effect." You might laugh, but listen closely next time, and you'll see I'm not too far off.

Calcium Channel Blockers

Calcium channel blockers include the drugs Diltiazem (Cardizem CD, Cardizem SR, Dilacor XR), Nifedipine (Procardia XL), and Verapamil (Calan, Calan SR, Isoptin, Isoptin SR, Verelan). These drugs slow the rate at which calcium passes to the contractile fibers of heart muscle and into the vessel walls. This action relaxes the vessels. Relaxed vessels allow the blood to flow more easily, thereby reducing blood pressure. Calcium channel blockers are used to treat chest pain (angina), high blood pressure, coronary artery disease, and irregular heartbeat (arrhythmia).

In 1995, the Public Citizen's Health Research Group filed a petition with the FDA to add a warning to the labeling of all calcium channel blockers. They cited observational studies that revealed that calcium channel blockers increase the risk of heart attack and death.[2] The FDA never added the warning.

Calcium channel blockers were put on the market without proper testing, according to Dr. Curt Furberg at the Wake Forest School of Medicine. For those who take them, there is not only an increase in strokes but a five-fold increase in the risk of heart attacks.[3]

The National Heart, Blood, and Lung Institute has warned doctors against the short-acting use of the calcium-channel blocker Procardia. The warning springs from the results of 16 studies involving over 8,000 patients. The risk of dying is doubled when a daily dose of 30–50 mg. is administered. The risk jumps to three times greater when 80 mg. a day is used.[4] But the maximum dose listed for Procardia is 180 mg. a day! I wonder how much *this* dose increases the risk of death? Death is a pretty scary side effect.

Why in the world are doctors still using calcium channel blockers for individuals with moderately elevated high blood pressure? The patient is probably more likely to die from taking the calcium channel blocker than they are from the moderately elevated blood pressure.

One study shows that those taking a calcium channel blocker are 60% more likely to have a heart attack than those taking a diuretic or beta blocker.[5,6]

Common side effects associated with calcium channel blockers are fatigue; flushing; swelling of the abdomen, ankles, or feet; and heartburn. Less common side effects are tachycardia (a racing heart), or bradycardia (a slow heart), shortness of breath, difficulty swallowing, dizziness, numbness in hands and feet, gastrointestinal bleeding, chest pains, jaundice, and fainting. Treatments combining calcium channel blockers and beta blockers increase the potential risk of side effects by 60%.[7]

Calcium channel blockers may also increase the risk of developing cancer.[8] Reports have demonstrated an increased risk of cancer among users of Verapamil, but it is too early to conclude that calcium channel blockers are associated with cancer.[9]

To add insult to injury, calcium channel blockers can make you stupid. Studies show that these drugs actually shrink the brain and decrease mental clarity.[10]

Beta Blockers

Commonly prescribed beta blockers include Atenolol (Tenoretic, Tenormin), Metoprolol (Lopressor, Toprol XL), Nadolol (Corgard), and Propranolol (Inderal). What these drugs block is the effects of adrenaline (and norepinephrine) on a cell's beta-receptors. In this way, they slow the nerve impulses that stimulate the heart, so the heart does not work as hard. Beta blockers are generally prescribed to treat high blood pressure (hypertension), congestive heart failure (CHF), abnormal heart rhythms (arrhythmias), and chest pain (angina). They are sometimes used in heart attack patients to prevent future attacks.

Beta blockers have several potential side effects, including congestive heart failure. I'm going to guess that if you knew a drug could cause your heart to die, you wouldn't take it. I know that I would say, "No thanks doc. I think I'll pass. You got any other options?"

Other side effects of beta blockers include shortness of breath, heart block, fatigue, lethargy, drowsiness, depression, insomnia, headaches, dizziness, tingling in the hands and feet, wheezing, bronchospasm, increased severity of asthma or chronic pulmonary obstructive disease, decreased sex drive, and muscle fatigue. And can you believe that beta blockers, used to treat the heart, actually reduce HDL (supposed "good" cholesterol) and increase LDL ("bad" cholesterol) and triglycerides in some folks?[11]

There have been periods in my practice where every new female patient I see is on a beta blocker. Is there some beta-blocker deficiency epidemic I haven't heard about? These beta blockers must be the drug du jour, since anyone with slight mitral valve prolapse, high blood pressure, or migraine headaches is placed on them. Beta blockers can be very valuable for a minority of patients. The majority, however, don't need them and suffer all sorts of health-robbing side effects. Patients who come to me on these medications often report that they just don't have any energy. That's probably because beta blockers depress your thyroid function, which causes fatigue, weight gain, and low moods.

One recent patient was on at least three medications to control her beta-blocker side effects: Lexapro as an antidepressant, Ambien to help her sleep, and a bronchial inhaler for asthma. Once she discontinued her medications with the help of her family doctor and substituted the nutritional supplements I recommended, her mitral valve prolapse and blood pressure returned to normal. The fatigue, depression, and breathing problems are slowly disappearing now that she is off her beta-blocking medication.

ACE Inhibitors

Commonly prescribed ACE inhibitors include Captopril (Capoten), Enalapril (Vasotec), and Lisinopril, (Prinivil, Zestril). These drugs, which inhibit the angiotensin-converting enzyme (ACE), decrease sodium and water retention, reduce blood pressure, improve cardiac output, and typically decrease heart size. They are used to treat congestive heart failure (CHF), arrhythmia, and hypertension. Following a heart attack, patients may be prescribed ACE inhibitors to prevent further damage to the heart. ACE inhibitors may also be prescribed for kidney problems associated with diabetes.

Potential side effects include a dry cough, gastrointestinal disturbances, numbness or tingling in the hands and feet, joint pain, fever, light-headedness, and fatigue.

These medications and the newer ACE II drugs appear to be the safest choice in cardiovascular-disease drugs. However, they can still cause serious adverse reactions, including bone marrow suppression and kidney disease.

One of my patients was taking an ACE drug and had been to several doctors about a persistent cough. The various doctors had prescribed asthma inhalers, prednisone dose packs, and antibiotics. When he discontinued his ACE drug, his cough disappeared. He was able to keep his blood pressure in check by using the natural supplements I recommended. You can find out how to do the same thing later in this book.

Angiotensin II–Receptor Blockers

When a patient is overwhelmed by the side effects of an ACE drug, his doctor might recommend one of these drugs, known as ARBs. They prevent angiotensin II from binding to its receptor site and so reduce arterial blood-vessel constriction (among other actions) and lower blood pressure. They are used to treat hypertension and CHF. ARBs include Diovan, Benicar, Micardis, Avapro, Cozaar, Teveten, and Atacand.

Potential side effects include headache, upper respiratory infection, cough, dizziness, sinusitis, throat inflammation, diarrhea, fatigue, back pain, viral infections, and abdominal pain.

Direct Vasodilators

Apresoline, Vasodilan, and Loniten (Minoxidil) are direct vasodilating drugs. Vasodilators open blood vessels by relaxing the muscular walls. These medications are used along with other cardiovascular drugs, because used alone they can cause increased heart rate, fluid retention, and swelling. Potential side effects include systemic lupus erythematosus (an inflammatory connective-tissue disease), headache, fatigue, low blood pressure, palpitations, increased heart rate, fluid retention, nasal congestion, weight gain, and increased body hair.

Antiarrhythmics

Cardiac glycosides are either obtained from the plants *digitalis purpurea* and *digitalis lanata* or are semisynthetic derivatives. These medications are commonly used for CHF, because they increase the force of cardiac contraction without significantly affecting other cardiovascular mechanisms. Cardiac glycosides include Digoxin, Digitoxin, Lanoxin, Purgoxin, and Crystodigin.

Digoxin causes over 28,000 cases of life-threatening or fatal adverse reactions each year. It has also been cited as overprescribed for seniors. One study revealed that 40% of those taking Digoxin were deriving no benefit from it. Digoxin toxicity occurs in one out of five individuals taking it. Toxic effects include hallucinations, nervousness, drowsiness, fatigue, loss of appetite, nausea, vomiting, abnormal heart rate, slow pulse rate, and problems with vision. (Could this be why your aunt Mary was recently diagnosed with senile dementia after years on Digoxin?) Digoxin levels must be properly monitored: too much leads to the symptoms above; too little can bring on heart failure.[12]

Cordarone is an antiarrhythmic used as a last resort to help regulate abnormal heart rhythms. Over 80% of those taking this medication will experience adverse, sometimes fatal, side effects. It can cause toxic reactions in the lungs, thyroid, and heart. Pulmonary toxicity (lung damage) was reported to have occurred in 10 of every 17 people who took the drug! Between 1 and 1.7% of those taken the drug die of lung complications.[13]

Class-I drugs used to help regulate heart rate include Quinidex, Norpace, Tambocor, Ethmozine, Procandid, Rythmol, Dura-Tabs, Duraquin, and Tonocard. They help slow the heart rate and decrease irregular heartbeats. These are heavy-duty drugs associated with a number of serious side effects. In the National Heart, Lung, and Blood Institute's Cardiac Arrhythmia Suppression Trial (CAST), nonfatal cardiac arrest were seen in 7.7% of those taking encainide (one of the antiarrhythmic Class-I drugs) and in only 3.3% in those taking a placebo. So when you take this drug, you've doubled your chances of such a heart attack.[14]

The FDA has placed a warning label on antiarrhythmics. Since they are associated with potentially fatal heart rhythms and there is no evidence to suggest they improve survival, only those individuals with life-threatening ventricular irregularities should be receiving them. Unfortunately, patients with non-life-threatening irregular atrial rhythms are commonly being prescribed these medications. This is a dangerous practice! Two antiarrhythmics—Tambacor and Enkaid—were shown to increase the risk of heart attack and death and were pulled off the market in 1989.

Potential side effects of antiarrhythmics include arrhythmia, heart block (heart attack), confusion, weakness, blurred vision, mental disturbances, and apathy.

Other antiarrhythmics include Quinagulate, Mexitil, Betapace, and Tikosyn.

Diuretics

Diuretics reduce edema (swelling) and lower blood pressure by reducing sodium and water retention. The three types of diuretics (thiazides, potassium-sparing diuretics, and high-loop diuretics) all work differently, but the goal is to lower blood pressure and/or heart fluid (in the case of CHF). These medications include Aldactone, Oretic, Euduron, Reneses, Hygroton, Bumex, Lasix, Anhydron, Diuril, Edecrin, Demadex, Dyrenium, Aldactone, Midamor, Zaroxolyn, and Lozol.

Lasix depletes vitamin B1 (thiamine), which is a crucial nutrient for the heart muscle. A B1 deficiency can cause any of the following: fatigue, mental confusion, depression, anxiety, upset stomach, and tingling in the hands and feet. It is estimated that 50% of elderly adults in the United States are deficient in vitamin B1. Now add Lasix, and you create another senile dementia case or someone who now needs an antidepressant medication. This scenario of chasing a side effect with another medication is all too common. But researchers found that when patients taking Lasix added 100 mg. of vitamin B1 daily, their heart function improved. Imagine that.[15]

Diuretics can cause excessive uric acid in the blood (gout), magnesium deficiency, potassium deficiency, electrolyte imbalance, muscle cramps, fatigue, headaches, lowered HDL, excessive sugar in the blood (diabetes), fever, rash, irregular menstrual cycles, impotence, and excessive urination and thirst.

The use of thiazide diuretics and potassium-sparing diuretics has demonstrated a modest increased risk of breast carcinoma, and the use of certain diuretics may increase the risk of breast carcinoma among older women.[16]

Diuretics have been shown to cause an 11-fold increase in diabetes.[17] Let me repeat this. Diuretics—yes, those little water pills—make you 11 times more likely to develop life-threatening diabetes! Obviously, my patients who tell me, "Doc, I'm just taking a little ol' water pill," don't know they may be setting themselves up for some serious health problems.

Aldactone is associated with several severe side effects, especially for individuals with kidney disease. It can cause kidney failure, muscle paralysis, and mental confusion in older adults. Dyrenium has been linked to kidney stones, kidney failure, and bone marrow suppression.[18] Diuretics also increase homocysteine, a chemical marker for risk of heart attack, stroke, Alzheimer's, depression, cancer, infertility, hypothyroid, diabetes, macular degeneration, and Parkinson's disease.[19,20,21] You'll read more about homocysteine later in this book.

Cholesterol-Lowering Drugs

The drugs most commonly used to lower total cholesterol, triglycerides, and LDL are the statin drugs, including lovastatin (Mevacor), pravastatin (Pravachol), simvastatin (Zocor), and atorvastatin (Lipitor). I discuss this class of drugs in chapter 8.

Bile-acid sequestrants are another class of drugs prescribed for reducing total cholesterol and LDL levels. These drugs include cholestyramine (LoCHOLEST, Questran) and colestipol (Colestid). Typically, gemfibrozil (Lopid), clofibrate (Atromid-S), and probucol (Lorelco) moderately reduce LDL levels.

A World Health Organization trial shows that use of Atromid-S actually increases mortality by 44%.[22] Animal studies show Questran causes intestinal cancer.[23] Several studies reveal that certain cholesterol-lowering drugs may increase the risk of cancer by one-third.[24]

Lopid does lower blood fats (triglycerides), but it doesn't lower cholesterol. "In fact, there is no proof that gemfibrozil has any health benefit, such as lowering the chance of having a heart attack, for most people with high blood cholesterol or fat levels."[25]

Potential side effects of bile-acid sequestrants include abdominal pain, acute appendicitis, atrial fibrillation, gallbladder disease, jaundice, dizziness, blurred vision, tingling in the hands or feet, headache, decreased sex drive, impotence, peripheral neuritis (pain), joint pain, altered taste, abnormal liver function tests, heart swelling, and rash.

You are more likely to die from taking these than you are from high triglycerides or cholesterol levels.

Other Potentially Dangerous Medications

Clonidine is used for high blood pressure. Missing only one or two doses of the drug can have serious consequences, including tremors, profuse sweating, and severely elevated blood pressure. Clonidine is also associated with severe depression. It shouldn't be used by anyone with a history of mood disorders.[26]

Coumadin is an anticoagulant medication used to prevent blood clots from forming within the arteries. It happens to be the same drug used to poison rats! It can cause several adverse reactions, all associated with internal bleeding (which is what kills the rats), including loss of consciousness, bloody or tarry stools, headaches, joint pain, muscle pain, constipation, abdominal pain, swelling in the ankles and feet, blue or purple toes, rashes, diarrhea, nausea, vomiting, unusual weight gain, nose bleeds, bleeding gums, and sores or white spots in the mouth.[27]

Trental is marketed as an effective drug to relieve leg cramps (known as intermittent claudication) caused by poor circulation. There is no proof or clinical data to support the claim that this medication improves blood circulation to the legs. According to the Hospital Pharmacy Therapeutics Committee at the University of California, San Francisco, Medical Center, studies are inconclusive as to the benefit of this drug.[28] This is also true for the drug Vasodilan, which is prescribed to increase the blood flow to the legs of those who suffer from muscle cramps. This medication is also associated with tingling in the hands and feet, nausea, chills, flushing, headache, and heart flutter.[29]

What About Aspirin?

The logic behind using aspirin to treat the heart is that it inhibits the formation of blood clots. But it does this by preventing the production of cyclooxygenase, an enzyme responsible for making prostaglandins. Prostaglandins are hormones that perform various bodily functions. Some cause platelets to become stickier and adhere to one another while attaching to arterial walls. However, other prostaglandins help prevent the platelets from attaching to one another. Thus, aspirin hinders the body's own natural self-regulating mechanisms.

This is similar to what happens when taking nonsteroidal anti-inflammatory drugs (NSAIDs). Aspirin is the original NSAID. It reduces inflammation by blocking prostaglandins 1, 2, and 3. The problem with this is that prostaglandins 1 and 3 are the body's own natural anti-inflammatory hormones; blocking them prevents the body from releasing its own natural pain-blocking chemicals.

There have been several studies investigating the role aspirin may play in reducing heart attacks. One in particular, The Aspirin Component of the Ongoing Physicians' Health Study, is cited by physician groups, the media, and of course, the drug companies who make aspirin.[30] This study involved 22,071 male physicians. Half of the study participants took Bufferin, and half took a placebo. The study shows that over a 4.8-year period, there were 44 deaths in the Bufferin group and 44 deaths in the placebo group. The Bufferin group did have fewer heart attacks (139 compared to 239) than the placebo group. Looking at the numbers above, we would conclude that taking Bufferin prevented 100 heart attacks. However, if we look at these numbers a little closer, you may choke on your aspirin.

If we take the 11,037 who took Bufferin and divide by 100 (the number who benefited from taking Bufferin) we see that .906% of those taking Bufferin benefited. This is of course less than 1%, a number not worth the fanfare it has received. So how is it that the researchers reported that those taking Bufferin had a 44%–47% reduction in heart attack risk? They took the 100 people who presumably didn't experience a heart attack because of taking Bufferin and divided it by the 239 who didn't take Bufferin and had a heart attack. This turns out to be 44%. That is some interesting analysis, to say the least. Researchers can do wonders with statistics!

An interesting finding that somehow wasn't revealed by this now famous study is that those taking Bufferin had a higher incidence of stroke (119), than those in the placebo group (98). Yet conventional doctors still advocate the use of aspirin for the prevention of stroke. If we were to use the same statistical parameters used by the authors of this study, we'd see that those taking Bufferin had a 21.4% increase in strokes! You won't hear that in the aspirin commercial.

Other less-quoted studies have evaluated the effectiveness of aspirin. A 1975 study involving one million American men and women showed no benefit at all.[31] The National Heart, Lung, and Blood Institute evaluated the effects of taking aspirin in a group of 4,524 participants who had had a heart attack. Half took aspirin and half took a placebo. The group who took aspirin had a 14.1% increase in heart attacks, while those taking a placebo had a 14.8% increase.[32] In 2003, a study linked low-dose aspirin use among elderly patients to decreased kidney function.[33]

Vioxx and Other NSAIDs

Merck has pulled the drug Vioxx off the market because a long-term clinical trial showed that some patients, after taking the drug for 18 months, developed serious heart problems. The data that ultimately persuaded the company to withdraw the drug indicated 15 cases of heart attack, stroke, or blood clots per thousand people each year over three years, compared with 7.5 such events per thousand patients taking a placebo. Internal memos show disagreement within the FDA over a study by one of its own scientists, Dr. David Graham, who estimated that Vioxx had been associated with more than 27,000 heart attacks or deaths linked to cardiac problems.

Studies have shown that Vioxx users had twice the number of heart attacks as those taking Naproxen, a COX-2 inhibitor. But these newer drugs, which block COX-2 enzymes, may still promote excessive blood-clot formation. It appears that COX-2 enzymes counteract some of the effects of COX-1 enzymes and so narrow the blood vessels. This narrowing then makes the blood more likely to clot.[34,35]

A person taking an NSAID—that includes aspirin—is seven times more likely to be hospitalized for gastrointestinal adverse affects. The FDA estimates that 200,000 cases of gastric bleeding occur annually, and that this leads to 10,000 to 20,000 deaths each year. NSAIDs can also cause high blood pressure. In fact, they more than double your risk.[36] Still, in one study, 41% of those who had recently started on medication to lower their blood pressure were also taking NSAIDs. Looks like nobody warned them.

The side effects associated with prescription medications are cause for rethinking how we treat CAD. Just as dangerous—if not more so—are the surgeries recommended for heart disease, as discussed in the next chapter.

Notes

1. November 2008 (Montvale, NJ: Thomson Healthcare).
2. C.D. Furberg, B.M. Patsy, and J.V. Meyer, "Nifedipine Dose-related Increase in Mortality in Patients with Coronary Heart Disease," *Circulation* 92 (1995): 1326–31.
3. ibid.
4. National Heart, Lung, and Blood Institute, "New Analysis Regarding the Safety of Calcium-channel Blockers," statement for health professionals (August 31, 1995).
5. C.D. Furberg et al., "Is it Safe to use Calcium Channel Blockers in Hypertension," *Lancet* 346 (1995): 586, 767–70.
6. B.M. Psaty et al., "The Risk of Myocardial Infarction Associated with Antihypertensive Drug Therapies," *Journal of the American Medical Association* 274 (1995): 620–5.
7. Milton Parker, "Second Generation Calcium Channel Blockers in the Treatment of Chronic Heart Failure: Are They Safe?" *New England Journal of Medicine* 320 (1989): 709–18.
8. M. Pahor et al., "Calcium-channel Blockade and Incidence of Cancer in Aged Populations," *Lancet* 348(9026) (1996): 493–7.
9. A.B. Beiderbeck-Noll et al., "Verapamil is Associated with an Increased Risk of Cancer in the Elderly: The Rotterdam Study," *European Journal of Cancer* 39(1) (2003): 98–105.
10. Sherry Rogers, *The Cholesterol Hoax* (Syracuse: Prestige, 2008).
11. N. Tanaka et al., "Effect of Chronic Administration of Propranolol on Lipoprotein Composition," *Metabolism* 25 (1976): 1071–5.
12. Sidney M. Wolfe, *Worst Pills Best Pills: A Consumer's Guide to Preventing Drug-Induced Death* (New York: Pocket, 1999).
13. Charles T. McGee, *Heart Frauds: Uncovering the Biggest Health Scam in History* (Colorado Springs: Piccadilly, 2001).
14. Sidney M. Wolfe, *Worst Pills Best Pills: A Consumer's Guide to Preventing Drug-Induced Death* (New York: Pocket, 1999).
15. H. Siegelmann et al., "Thiamine Deficiency in Patients with Congestive Heart Failure Receiving Long-term Furosemide Therapy: a Pilot Study," *American Journal of Medicine* 91 (1991): 151–5.
16. C.I. Li et al., "Relation Between Use of Antihypertensive Medications and Risk of Breast Carcinoma Among Women Ages 65–79 years," *Cancer* 98(7) (2003):1504–13.
17. Peter T. Sawick, correspondence, *British Medical Journal* 308 (1994):855.
18. *Physicians' Desk Reference* (Montvale, NJ: Medical Economics Data Production, 1995), 1851–54.
19. S. Westphal et al., "Antihypertensive Treatment and Homocysteine Concentrations," *Metabolism* 52(3) (March 2003): 261–3.
20. N. Chen et al., "Physiological Concentrations of Homocysteine Inhibit the Human Plasma GSH Peroxidase that Reduces Organic Hydroperoxides," *Journal of Laboratory and Clinical Medicine* 136(1) (2000): 58–65.

21. Sherry Rogers, *The High Blood Pressure Hoax* (Syracuse: Prestige, 2005).
22. J.F. Fries et al., "A Co-operative Trial in the Primary Prevention of Ischemic Heart Disease Using Clofibrate," *British Heart Journal* 40 (1978): 1069–1118.
23. *Physicians' Desk Reference,* (Montvale, NJ: Medical Economics Data Production, 1995), 710–712.
24. ibid., 1851–54.
25. Sidney M. Wolfe, *Worst Pills Best Pills: A Consumer's Guide to Preventing Drug-Induced Death* (New York: Pocket, 1999).
26. ibid.
27. ibid.
28. Pharmacy and Therapeutics Forum, 1987:4. Cited in *Worst Pills Best Pills.*
29. A.G. Gilman et al., eds. *The Pharmalogical Basis of Therapeutics,* 8th edition (New York: Pergamon, 1990): 226–7.
30. Steering Committee on the Physicians' Health Study Research Group, "Final Report on the Aspirin Component of the Ongoing Physicians' Health Study," *New England Journal of Medicine* 321(3) (1989): 129–35.
31. E.C. Hammond and L. Garfinkel, "Aspirin and Coronary Heart Disease: Findings of a Prospective Study," *British Medical Journal* (1975): 269–271.
32. Aspirin Myocardial Infarction Study Research Group, "A Randomized Trail of Aspirin in Persons Recovered From Myocardial Infarction," *Journal of the American Medical Association* 243 (1980): 661–669.
33. R. Segal et al., "Early and Late Effects of Low-Dose Aspirin on Renal Function in Elderly Patients," *American Journal of Medicine* 115 (October 15, 2003): 462–6.
34. David Lincoln Nelson, "Dr. Nelson's Non-Steroidal Anti-Inflammatory Drugs and Cox-2 Inhibitor Page," (April 18, 2006), www.davidlnelson.md/COX2Inhibitors.htm.
35. J. Zhang et al., "Adverse Effects of Cyclooxygenase 2 Inhibitors on Renal and Arrhythmia Events: Meta-analysis of Randomized Trials," *Journal of the American Medical Association* 13 (2006): 1619–32.
36. Peter M. Brooks and Richard O. Day, "Nonsteroidal Anti-Inflammatory Drugs: Differences and Similarities," *New England Journal of Medicine* 324(24) (1991): 1716–25.

3

What You Must Know About Heart Surgery

CONVENTIONAL MEDICAL TREATMENTS for advanced coronary disease includes bypass surgery, balloon angioplasty, heart transplants, and cardiac catheterization. Although surgery is sometimes necessary and can help save lives, it is not without considerable risk. Surgery should always be the last option, never the first; a large number of heart surgeries performed could have been avoided. (A conservative estimate reveals that six million unnecessary operations occur each year in the United States. For instance, 20,000 normal appendixes are removed each year.)[1]

BYPASS SURGERY

It's no better than placebo. Bypass and angioplasty surgeries have never been proven to be more effective than a placebo. To be fair, *most* medical therapies have never been proven effective. The prestigious British magazine *New Scientist* announced that 80% of all medical procedures in use have never been scientifically proven.[2] But when it comes to heart surgery, even the tests used to diagnose whether the surgery is needed have been shown to be largely meaningless, and experience has played this truth out.

For instance, one of the first surgeries to be performed for angina (chest pain) was a procedure where heart surgeons tied off the internal mammary arteries. The reasoning was that if these two arteries running along the rib cage were tied off, more blood would be available to the heart, and this would relieve the chest pain. Several studies showed that 36% of patients receiving this surgery later reported themselves as pain-free. Consequently, the procedure became very popular and was hailed as a major breakthrough for relieving angina pain. However, a funny thing happened one day. A certain prominent cardiac surgeon, in his rush to sew up his patient, forgot to tie off the arteries. The patient awoke from surgery and reported that he was free of pain! The patient had been cured by the greatest healer of all—the placebo response!

A placebo response occurs when a sugar pill is given (or a sham surgery performed) and the patient gets well on his own. (You see, the greatest healer resides within you.) Once doctors found out that internal mammary surgery was no better than placebo, the procedure was abandoned as useless.

Other fad heart surgeries have been tried over the years. Many were advocated as the new treatment of choice, until they too were exposed as no better than placebo. This includes one surgical procedure in which surgeons blew talcum powder onto the pericardium sac in hopes that this would stimulate new blood-vessel growth. Amazingly, patients reported dramatic relief from their persistent angina. Of course, once again, this procedure was found to be no better than placebo and was abandoned.

However, a new surgical procedure known as coronary artery bypass grafting (CABG) came on the market in the late 1960s, and it spread like wildfire. In CABG (sometimes casually called "cabbage"), the surgeon reroutes, or bypasses, blood around clogged arteries to improve blood flow and increase oxygen to the heart. To accomplish this, a vein is taken from another part of the patient's body and inserted around the clogged artery. To keep the patient alive during the operation, a bypass pump takes the blood from the veins entering the heart, puts oxygen into it, and pumps it into the arteries.

The procedure, known to most as "bypass surgery," lives on today, despite never undergoing placebo-controlled studies. Conventional medicine continues to ridicule alternative therapies for not having double-blind placebo studies (although many do) to prove their effectiveness. Yet the highly dangerous bypass surgery has never been tested to see whether it is more effective than placebo.

The placebo response is quite useful; it's cured many patients even without their knowledge! Many antidepressant medications, for instance, have been shown to be no more than 25% more effective than a placebo, yet millions of Americans take them and report feeling better because of them.[3] The placebo response has been observed in the treatment of hypertension, angina, type-2 diabetes, intermittent claudication, and many other diseases. So, how do we know for sure that today's surgical procedures for heart disease are any more effective than a placebo? We just don't.

When the Office of Technology Assessment was commissioned by the U.S. Congress to review the case for surgery in the treatment of coronary artery disease, it was not greatly impressed. A panel of government consultants, which included leading academicians from the nation's most prestigious medical schools, reported to Congress:

> For more than half a century, surgeons have believed that an efficacious surgical approach to coronary artery disease is possible. Prior to the modern bypass operation, five different operations were developed and advocated enthusiastically. Although all five operations were ultimately abandoned as of no value, initially they were alleged to be efficacious, with reports in the medical literature claiming 'objective' evidence of benefits.

Noting that "coronary bypass surgery seems to give excellent symptomatic relief from angina pectoris…but the improvement diminishes with time," the government panel of experts cautioned that there was an historical lesson to be heeded, pointing out that "the possible placebo effect [of bypass surgery] needs to be kept in mind because: the initial results are similar to previous operations; nonsurgical treatment also produces good results; and, the methods of evaluation of symptomatic relief are experiential."[4]

The chief of cardiology at the Montreal Heart Institute, Dr. Lucien Campeau, is a cardiovascular specialist who suspects that long-term relief of angina pain results from what he calls a "pain-denial placebo effect." Dr. Campeau came to this conclusion after studying 235 patients three years after their bypass operations, discovering that even in cases where grafts had reclosed, patients reported being improved or angina-free.[5]

Now, no one is claiming that bypass surgery doesn't do something for patients in pain. There is no doubt that bypass surgery relieves angina 75% of the time, and for those with persistent angina, relief is a welcomed outcome. But are the results long-lasting? Not hardly. Somewhere between 30% and 50% of patients undergoing bypass surgery will have recurring symptoms within one year![6]

Of course, it's tough to prove the placebo effect with surgery. No one wants to possibly undergo a fake surgical procedure. It's generally considered inhumane. Therefore, very few surgical procedures have ever been tested against placebo. However, one popular surgical procedure *was* tested, and it failed.

An estimated 12% of Americans ages 65 and older have osteoarthritis of the knee. A recent study that evaluated the effectiveness of knee surgery showed that surgery was no better than placebo. In this case, the placebo was a fake operation described as "a sham" by Dr. Baruch Brody, an ethicist at Baylor University who helped design the study.[7]

Dr. Thomas Preston, professor of medicine at University of Washington, Seattle, writes that "except for a well-defined minority of patients, and in most cases, cabbage surgery…is no better than placebo." He is rather to the point: "Coronary bypass surgery is one of the most over-hyped and over-utilized surgeries in America!"[8]

It doesn't extend life. Recently, a good friend of mine was rushed to his local emergency room with chest pain. Before he knew it, he was "in the system," as he called it. They started him on medications and quickly arranged for an angiogram. Sure enough, even though he had never smoked, had normal blood pressure and cholesterol levels, and had never before had chest pains, the test suggested that he had two blocked arteries. The surgeon on call suggested surgery immediately. The surgeon did not discuss any other options, nor did he address any of the potential risks associated with the surgery. A small risk known as *death* should have been mentioned, but wasn't.

My friend, in a state of shock, confusion, and severe medication fog, asked if he could go home and think about it for a few days and perhaps get a second opinion. The surgeon was not too accommodating; his reply went something like this:

> Mr. Murdock, you have two blocked arteries. These arteries are choking off the blood supply to your heart. If you don't have surgery, you'll have a heart attack and die. Why, I don't even know if you can make it home or not, much less have a day or two to think about it. You are a walking time bomb.

Pressured by his understandably worried wife, my friend had the surgery performed that day. Fortunately, he had a technically gifted surgeon, and his operation went well. But nothing compared to the "pain" he felt several weeks later when he had the chance to discuss his ordeal with me. I presented him with some of the material from this book, and he found out that neither of the arteries involved had been more than 40% blocked. Nor did they involve the left ventricle function (more about this below). I was able to refer him to a more enlightened medical doctor who helped my friend wean off his heart medications. I'm happy to report that since he has been following my advice, he has lost 20 pounds, is off all prescription medications, walks an hour each day, takes the appropriate nutritional supplements, and looks 10 years younger.

Being called "a walking time bomb" is sobering stuff, no doubt. But is there any truth to the statement? A Veterans Administration study compared 486 heart patients who were divided into two groups, those who did and those who did not have bypass surgery. At the end of eleven years, there was no difference in survival rates.[9] This study sent shock waves through the cardiac community. They had been advocating bypass surgery as a means of increasing lifespan and now were faced with a study that clearly showed this was not the case. Bypass surgery does help angina, but it doesn't ensure that you'll live any longer. Heart surgeons have known *this* since the 1970s, when a series of highly regarded studies showed that coronary bypass surgery, while relieving angina, didn't improve survival except in patients with severe coronary disease or those with left ventricular blockage.[10]

Another study involving 14 major heart hospitals around the world showed that one-third of all heart bypass surgeries were unnecessary and actually increased the risk of death. And one-third of these patients would have lived longer if they had received drug therapy instead of surgery.[11]

The National Institutes of Health has estimated that 90% of Americans who undergo bypass surgery receive no benefits![12] Yes. You read that right. No benefit. In fact, a Swedish study revealed that 12% of those undergoing bypass suffered obvious brain damage, including strokes.[13]

Perhaps the most definitive study to date, The Coronary Artery Surgery Study (CASS) showed that these teaching hospitals, where bypass was being *taught to other physicians,* had a death rate from bypass surgery between 1% and 9% percent. And these folks are the experts.[16]

Let's see, my doctor recommends "lifesaving" heart bypass surgery. However, I'm more likely to live if I don't have surgery than if I do. I probably don't even need the surgery, it holds a 10% risk of death, and I could suffer brain damage? Yes, that is exactly what the leading medical journals are saying. Obviously, medical doctors are either not reading these journals or are choosing to ignore their findings.

There are other serious risks. Death isn't the only possible side effect of bypass surgery. It is certainly no assurance against a heart attack, given that 5% to 10% of those undergoing bypass surgery experience a heart attack immediately following the operation, according to the New York Heart Association, brain damage is another common occurrence that can result in permanent neurological or cognitive disturbances. Mental disturbances (for as long as five years) are seen in up to 53% of patients undergoing bypass surgery.[17]

Do women fare any better than men in bypass surgery? No. In fact, women are 77% more likely to die from bypass surgery than men are. Plainly, women should especially avoid bypass surgery. It is certainly more dangerous than their diagnosis of heart disease.[18]

There are safer, better options. Before folks with chronic angina agree to bypass surgery, they should be made aware that the *New England Journal of Medicine* has stated that 75% of angina patients' pain can also be relieved with nonsurgical therapy.[19] And given all risks we've discussed, prescription medication for the management of angina should be appealing. The good news is that the percentage of those who improve on the medication is the same as those who improve after the surgery. [20] Consider the testimony of patients whose vein grafts have ceased to function after their operation. More than a hundred such cases have been identified. Yet before finding out that their bypasses were again blocked, these patients reported the *same* amelioration of symptoms as those who had had successful operations.[21]

The Money Behind the Surgery

Bypass surgery is a multibillion-dollar industry, with approximately 467,000 bypasses and 1,244,000 percutaneous coronary interventions (PCIs) performed in the United States in 2003 alone. At an average cost of about $45,000 each, bypass surgeries and the ancillary medical costs associated with them add up to billions of dollars for the American health-care system: an estimated $12 to $20 billion a year.[22] These surgeries are major revenue producers for hospitals, cardiologist, anesthesiologists, surgical nurses, and of course cardiac surgeons, who make between $3,000 and $6,000 for each surgery. It is not unusual for these surgeons to do over 150 bypasses a year.

Entire medical wings have been funded by the big business of grafting leg veins and rerouting blood.[23] I can imagine that these folks get a little nervous when studies don't show that bypass surgery is needed in 90% of the cases and worse, that it may cause more harm than good.[24]

Interestingly, individuals on Medicaid (which pays far less than does private insurance) are 80% less likely to be recommended for an angiogram. Patients with private insurance were also 40% more likely to receive bypass surgery than those on Medicaid.[25]

In Europe, doctors are paid purely on a salary basis. Not surprisingly, European doctors recommend bypass surgery 75% less often than do their American counterparts.[26] Maybe doctors in Europe don't see as many cardiac patients as doctors in the United States. I wish this were true, but the fact is they see just as many heart disease patients as American doctors do. Perhaps they just see them with both eyes open.

Now, before my neighbors, who happen to be cardiac surgeons, ostracize me from future block parties, I want to go on record as saying that these folks deserve to be paid well for their skills and that most cardiac surgeons, like most other doctors, do truly care about their patients. Cardiac surgeons are some of the most dedicated, hardworking, and highly skilled professionals in the field of medicine. However, medical studies reveal the following about heart surgery: it is not needed 90% of the time, it causes mental damage in a majority of patients, it triggers heart attacks in 10% of patients, it fails to produce long-term relief, it doesn't extend life (except in a small minority of patients), and it is implicated in many of the deaths of heart patients. The National Heart and Lung Institute reported that the risk of death following coronary bypass surgery is between 1%–4% in the best case and 10%–15% in the worst case.[27]

Angioplasty

Angioplasty is a surgical procedure used to widen blocked arteries of the heart. Percutaneous transluminal coronary angioplasty (PTCA or *balloon* angioplasty) involves threading a catheter with an inflatable balloon-like tip through the arteries to the blocked area. The balloon is inflated, thereby widening the arterial channel, flattening the fatty deposits, and allowing more blood to reach the heart muscle. Over 700,000 angioplasty surgeries are performed each year in the United States.

In *laser* angioplasty a laser-tipped catheter is guided to the blockage, and the laser is used to destroy the plaque buildup within the artery.

In *stent* angioplasty, a tiny metal stent, attached to the tip of the catheter, is inserted into a clogged blood vessel. The catheter is then threaded up the blocked vessel (usually coronary arteries), and the stent is strategically placed in order to prop open the block vessel. Over one million Americans undergo stent therapy each year, and researchers have found that the procedure does increase blood flow and reduce chest pain. However, the results are *no better* than drug therapy alone, according to research published in April 2007 in the New England Journal of Medicine.[28]

The big difference between stents and drugs is the cost. Angioplasty with stents generally costs about $25,000. The drug-coated stents cost an additional $2,200. Stent angioplasty generates some $3 billion annually for Boston Scientific and Johnson and Johnson. So the results mentioned above triggered, of course, a barrage of public-relations "spin" from these companies. Even though the study showed that those taking traditional cardiac drugs fared just as well as those having stent therapy—7 out of 10 in both groups reported less chest pain—David Kandzari of Johnson and Johnson insisted that "both should be used." Now why on earth might he say that?

Though angioplasty might help relieve pain, its effects are not always permanent. They often don't last even a year. From 50% to 60% of patients having angioplasty for leg arteries have blockages return within nine months. And 20–30% of those having angioplasty for heart arteries will have to have the surgery again within nine months.

Studies routinely show that almost 10% of those undergoing angioplasty will have a heart attack, need additional surgery, or die immediately following surgery.[29] Blood clots form in up to 29% of those receiving medicated stent therapy. For certain heart-attack patients, these clots increase the risk of death within 24 months of the procedure for 400%, according to recent research presented at the meeting of the European Society of Cardiology in Vienna.[30] Patients are instructed to use Coumadin to counter this risk. I'm not a fan of this drug, as I make clear in chapter 2. I recommend my patients avoid rat poison and instead use the natural clot-busting supplement, nattokinase.

And although the death rate for angioplasty is rather low compared to bypass surgery (2% compared to 9–10%), survival rates of those undergoing angioplasty are only 3% better than for those not having the surgery. Keep in mind that the annual mortality for patients with two- and three-vessel disease who are treated conservatively with appropriate medication is less than 1% per year. For patients with a disease of all three coronary arteries who undergo coronary angioplasty, the annual mortality rate is 4.2 %. [31] In fact, one study shows that only 13% of angioplasty patients with two or more risk factors (smoking, obesity, sedentary lifestyle, etc.) were still alive five years after their surgery.[32]

Angiograms

The angiogram—the test to determine if someone needs bypass surgery—is not without controversy either. Over one million angiograms are performed each year, costing over $10 billion. These tests use a long, thin catheter with a tiny camera for the purpose of observing arterial blockages. The catheter is inserted into the femoral artery (in the groin area) and then threaded up the aorta to the heart. A dye is injected, which allows x-ray monitoring of its progress as it flows through the arteries and heart. The first angiogram was performed in 1963.

In 1976, the Harvard Medical School Office of Information Technology performed a review of angiograms. Four angiogram experts were asked to participate. Some had been interpreting angiograms for over nine years, and each had read a minimum of 1,500 angiograms and were responsible for teaching other doctors the technique. These experts all separately reviewed the same angiograms, and then their interpretations were compared. The study found that wide differences in the doctors' interpretations were common. One expert read an area of artery as being 100% blocked. Another interpreted the same area of artery to be 100% blockage free![33]

Even if blockages are accurately interpreted, the blockage percentage doesn't necessarily indicate a need for surgery. One study showed that the severity of the blockage has no bearing on blood flow! Measuring the blood flow in 44 blocked arteries as demonstrated by angiogram, researchers found that the heart arteries with up to 96% blockage had the swiftest blood flow. This same study showed that some arteries with only a 40% blockage had a reduced blood flow. The authors concluded that the blockages found on heart catheterization do not correlate with blood-flow restrictions.[34]

Another study (never published) was presented at the American Heart Association in 1979. Thirty previously read angiograms were circulated among the same experts who had read them the first time. The doctors' interpretations *significantly disagreed* with their previous readings 32% of the time.[35]

In another study, readings of the heart were taken using Doppler technology while the chest was open during bypass surgery. The authors cited the Doppler readings as accurate but had a very different opinion about the previous angiograms:

> The physiologic effects of the majority of coronary obstructions can not be determined accurately by conventional angiographic approaches. The results of these studies should be profoundly disturbing to all physicians who have relied on the coronary arteriogram to provide accurate information regarding the physiologic consequences of individual coronary stenosis.[36]

The authors of this study were being tactful; I won't be. Angiograms are worthless. Their inaccurate results are dangerously misleading to doctors and patients. And they are overused anyway. One study showed that 80% of those scheduled for angiogram were getting one unnecessarily, according to other testing procedures.[37]

Despite these studies being in peer-reviewed medical journals, nothing has changed. Like many medical procedures, the rituals of heart surgery and angiograms are venerated as valuable despite evidence to the contrary for most patients. If you are a heart patient and a cardiac surgeon recommends a surgical procedure where he intends to cut through your breast bone with a power saw, hook you up to a machine while your heart stops beating, remove a piece of vein from your leg, produce mental deterioration in your brain (53% chance), increase your chance of heart attack by up to 10%, and possibly bring on your premature death, he better have a dog-and-pony show that demonstrates the need for this surgery. One faulty angiogram, considered meaningless by some experts, certainly shouldn't be enough to convince you.

Just consider their rationale: find the blocked artery and reroute the plumbing around it (or inflate it with a balloon or metal stent) for increased blood flow. What about the other 60,000 miles of arteries and veins just waiting to block? The patch-and-reroute mentality, analogous to repairing rusty pipes, reveals how short-sighted conventional medicine has been in its approach to heart disease.

When *Is* Surgery Needed?

As you've already read, studies clearly show that in general, those who elect not to have heart surgery live as long, if not longer, than those who do have surgery.[38] However, there are situations where heart surgery is worth the risk. But the determining factor has little to do with how many blockages are present, or the percentages of their extent. The body has its own way of dealing with blockages. When arteries become blocked, alternative courses of blood flow are created through other arteries.

The CASS study demonstrates that, because of the body's ability to compensate for blockages, surgery is simply not necessary when the left ventricle is functioning above 40%. However, once the left ventricle's function goes below 40%, surgery does in fact increase life span.

Therefore, the most important factor in determining if someone truly could benefit from a bypass or angioplasty surgery is how well the left ventricle is performing, not the degree or number of arterial blockages. To put it clinically, surgery is only helpful when the heart's ejection fraction of the left ventricle is less than 40%. Sadly, 90% of all bypass surgeries (including all their risks) are performed on men and women with ejection fractions above 40%.[39]

"What Should I Do?"

Plainly, it is *best* to keep your cardiovascular system as healthy as you can with diet, supplementation, and when necessary, prescription medications. Surgery should be your last resort and then only when the left ventricular ejection fraction is less than 40%. If, heaven forbid, you do find yourself being rushed to the emergency room with chest pains, try to remain calm and keep your wits about you.

Don't let the doctors scare you into doing anything you don't want to do. Gather all the information. Ask for all your options. Insist on an echocardiogram or a nuclear medicine scan to see if you do truly need surgery. Find out what your left ventricular ejection rate is. If it is greater than 40%, know that studies show your survival without the surgery is as good, if not better, than if you have the surgery.

Realize the medical establishment is going to do everything in their power to encourage you toward the surgery. They can't just do "nothing": They don't want to get sued any more than you want to die. Money and politics aside, your doctor has likely bought into the idea that surgery is the answer. She isn't going to let you off the hook without some serious mental duress.

Remember, their position is non-negotiable. They believe wholeheartedly (no pun intended) in what they do. If they didn't, they wouldn't be able to sleep at night. Heart surgeons are brilliant, well-meaning folks, but just because they believe (and that's all it is—a belief) that surgery is the only option doesn't mean you have to believe it. Get all the facts, and then make your decision.

I recommend the following tests for determining your risk of cardiovascular disease.

- **echocardiogram.** This noninvasive ultrasound test records and measures the beating heart, its blood flow, and the thickness of the heart's chambers.
- **nuclear stress test.** The Rolls Royce of stress tests and superior to ordinary EKG, a nuclear stress test uses a sophisticated computerized camera to monitor your heart while you exercise.
- **64-slice coronary CT scan.** This noninvasive procedure will one day replace the antiquated and flawed coronary angiogram.
- **electron beam computerized tomography.** The EBT measures hardened plaque in coronary arteries.

Just as important as coronary tests are blood tests. I'll have more to say about these later in the book, but here is a quick-reference list.

- **high sensitivity C-reactive protein** (hsCrP)
- **fibrinogen**
- **ferriten** (Too much iron doubles your risk of heart attack.)
- **LDL**
- **lipoprotein A** (Lp[a]) (Elevated levels are a warning sign and can lead to blood clots forming on top of existing plaque.)
- **HDL** (Low levels of this good cholesterol are more dangerous than elevated total cholesterol.)
- **triglycerides** (blood fats)
- **homocysteine** (marker for heart disease risk)
- **vitamin E** (The status of this important antioxidant is more accurate than cholesterol levels.)
- **RBC magnesium**
- **CoQ10** (Low levels of coenzyme q10 suggest cardiovascular disease.)

A **cardio/ion panel** is *the test* for those who want to know their cardiovascular risk status and—just as importantly—what to do to correct any biochemical deficiencies or dysfunctions. It measures HDL, LDL, Lp(a), triglycerides, homocysteine, fibrinogen, CRP, 8-OhdG, lipid peroxides, insulin, testosterone, and RBC nutrients—magnesium, vitamin E, fatty acids, CoQ10, heavy metals, organic acids, and amino acids. For a list of doctors who order this test, see "Laboratories" in the appendix. If you have a hard time finding a doctor who will order the test for you, feel free to call my clinic at 1-888-884-9577 or visit www.treatingandbeating.com and click on "Lab Test Finder."

Genova Diagnostics offers a similar (although not quite as extensive) profile known as Cardiovascular Comprehensive 2.0. See the appendix for their information.

The best defense, of course, is a good offense. In the next few chapters, we'll look at ways to help you prevent a heart attack and reverse the effects of coronary artery disease. Let's spend some time learning about the amazing cardiovascular system.

Notes

1. Stephen Fulder, *How to Survive Medical Treatment: A Holistic Guide to Avoiding the Risks and Side-Effects of Conventional Medicine* (London: Century Hutchinson, 1987).
2. *New Scientist* (September 17, 1994), 23.
3. I. Kirsh and G. Sapirstein, "Listening to Prozac but Hearing Placebo: A Meta-analysis of Antidepressant Medications," *Prevention and Treatment* 1(0002a) (1998).
4. Congress of the United States, Office of Technology Assessment, "Assessing the Efficacy and Safety of Medical Technologies," publication 052-003-00593-0 (Washington D.C.: Government Printing, 1978).
5. Elmer M. Cranton, "What You Should Know About Bypass Surgery and Angioplasty," web article (2001), www.drcranton.com/chelation/angioplasty.htm.
6. I.C. Gilchrist et al., "Temporal Spectrum of Ischemic Complications with Percutaneous Coronary Intervention: The Esprit Experience," *Lancet* 356 (2000): 2037–44.
7. Gina Kolata, "A Knee Surgery for Arthritis is Called Sham," *New York Times* accessed through the University of British Columbia at www.econ.ubc.ca/evans/384nyt.pdf.
8. Thomas Preston, "Marketing an Operation: Coronary Artery Bypass Surgery," *Journal of Holistic Medicine* 7(1) (1985): 5–15.
9. R.J. Luchi et al., "Comparison of Medical and Surgical Treatment for Unstable Angina Pectoris," *New England Journal of Medicine* 316(16) (1987): 977–84.
10. P. MacDonald, D. Johnstone, and K. Rockwood, "Coronary Bypass Surgery for Elderly Patients: Is Our Practice Based on Evidence or Faith?" *Canadian Medical Association Journal* 162(7) (2000).
11. A.F. Parisi, E.D. Folland, and P. Hartigan, "A Comparison of Angioplasty with Medical Therapy in the Treatment of Single-vessel Coronary Artery Disease," *New England Journal of Medicine* 326 (1992): 10–16.
12. Lynn McTaggart, *What Doctors Don't Tell You: The Truth About The Dangers of Modern Medicine* (New York: Avon, 1998).
13. A. Torkel, *Scandinavia Journal of Thoracic and Cardiovascular Surgery* (supplement) 15 (1974).
14. Harold and Arline Brecher, *Forty Something Forever* (Herndon, VA: Health Savers, 2000), 6.
15. ibid.
16. M.F. Newman et al., "Longitudinal Assessment of Neurocognitive Function After Coronary-artery Bypass Surgery," *New England Journal of Medicine* 344 (6) (2001):395–402.
17. Harold and Arline Brecher, *Forty Something Forever* (Herndon, VA: Health Savers, 2000).
18. ibid.

19. William E. Boden, "Optimal Medical Therapy With or Without PCI for Stable Coronary Disease," *New England Journal of Medicine,* web article, published at www.nejm.org on March 26, 2007.
20. ibid.
21. Elmer M. Cranton, "What You Should Know About Bypass Surgery and Angioplasty."
22. American Heart Association, "Angioplasty More Cost-effective Than Bypass Surgery for Some Men," journal report (September 11, 2006), www.americanheart.org/presenter.jhtml?identifier=3041920.
23. Note: According to the American Heart Association, there were 1,297,000 angiograms performed in 2004 at an average cost of $10,880 per procedure. This resulted in 427,000 bypass surgeries at an average cost of $83,919 each and 664,000 percutaneous transluminal (balloon) coronary angioplasties (PTCAs) at an average of $38,203 each. The total bill in 2004 was $12–20 billion. The total annual cost of cardiovascular disease in the United States, including medications and disability, is approximately $283 billion per year. Source: "Heart Disease and Stroke Statistics 2007 Update," *Circulation Journal of the American Heart Association,* http://circ.ahajournals.org/cgi/content/full/CIRCULATIONAHA.106.179918.
24. M.B Wenneker, "The Association of Payer with Utilization of Cardiac Procedures in Massachusetts" *Journal of the American Medical Association* 264 (1990): 1255–1260.
25. Charles T. McGee, *Heart Frauds* (Colorado Springs: HealthWise, 2001), 33.
26. L.A. Cobb et al., "The Veterans Study," *New England Journal of Medicine* 311 (1977): 1311–1339.
27. Elmer Cranton, *Bypassing Bypass Surgery* (Charlottsville: Hampton Roads, 2001), 237.
28. W. Boden et al., "Optimal Medical Therapy With or Without PCI for Stable Coronary Disease," *New England Journal of Medicine* 356(15) (2007): 1503–16.
29. Charles T. McGee, *Heart Frauds* (Colorado Springs: HealthWise, 2001), 45.
30. P.G. Steg, "Increased All-cause Mortality at Two-year Follow-up After PCI with Drug-Eluting Stents vs. Bare Metal Stents in Acute Coronary Syndromes: The GRACE Registry," Presented at the European Society of Cardiology Congress (September 1, 2007), Vienna.
31. E.L. Hannan et al., "Three-year Survival After Coronary Artery Bypass Graft Surgery and Percutaneous Transluminal Coronary Angioplasty," *Journal of the American College of Cardiology* 33 (1999): 63–72.
32. W. Hueb, "Two- to Eight-year Survival Rates in Patients Who Refused Coronary Artery Bypass Grafting," *American Journal of Cardiology* 68 (1989): 939–950.
33. C.W. White et al., "Does Visual Interpretation of Coronary Angiogram Predict the Physiologic Importance of a Coronary Stenosis," *New England Journal of Medicine* 310 (1984): 819–824.
34. ibid.

35. ibid.
36. CASS Principle Investigators and Their Associates, "Coronary Artery Surgery (CASS): A Randomized Trial of Coronary Artery Bypass Surgery," *Circulation* 68 (1983): 939–950.
37. S. Paulin, "Assessing the Severity of Coronary Lesions with Angiography," *New England Journal of Medicine* 316(22) (1987): 1405–7.
38. C.M. Winslow et al., "The Appropriateness of Performing Coronary Bypass Surgery," *Journal of the American Medical Association* 260 (1988): 505.
39. C.M. Grondin et al., "Discrepancies Between Cineangiographic and Postmortem Findings in Patients with Coronary Artery Disease and Recent Myocardial Revascularization," *Circulation* 49 (1974): 703–8.

4

The Amazing Cardiovascular System

REMEMBER EIGHTH-GRADE HEALTH CLASS? Well, consider this chapter a refresher course. The cardiovascular (circulatory) system is made up of the heart, blood vessels, and lymphatics. It's responsible for delivering life-sustaining oxygen and nutrients to every cell in the body. It removes metabolic waste products and helps carry hormones from one part of the body to another. And this *will* be on the test: arteries carry blood away from the heart, veins carry blood to the heart, and capillaries (tiny blood vessels) deliver blood to the tissues.

THE HEART

The heart is a small muscular organ about the size of a human fist. It only weighs about 11 ounces, but the heart's structure makes it an efficient, unceasing pump. From the point of development through the moment of death, the heart pumps. Therefore, it has to be strong. The average cardiac muscle contracts and relaxes about 70 to 80 times per minute.

The heart beats more than 100,000 times and pumps nearly 2,000 gallons of blood throughout the body's circulatory system every day. The vast network of blood vessels, including arteries, capillaries, and veins, is over 60,000 miles long—more than twice the distance around the earth.[1]

Chambers and Valves

The heart is really two separate pumps divided into two chambers each. The top two chambers are known as the left and right atria. The bottom two chambers are known as the left and right ventricles.

The **right atrium** pumps blood down to the right ventricle. From there, the **right ventricle** pumps blood to the lungs.

The **left atrium** pumps blood down to the left ventricle. From there, the **left ventricle** pumps blood to the rest of the body.

The heart contracts in two stages. In the first stage, the right and left atria contract at the same time, pumping blood to the right and left ventricles. Then the ventricles contract together to pump blood out of the heart.

Each chamber has a one-way valve at its exit that prevents blood from flowing backwards.

The **tricuspid valve** connects the right atrium to the right ventricle.

The **pulmonary valve** connects the right ventricle to the pulmonary artery.

The **mitral valve** connects the left atrium to the left ventricle.

The **aortic valve** connects the left ventricle to the aorta.

Circulation

This is how this system of pumps and valves distributes the oxygen we need. Used, oxygen-poor blood enters the heart through the right atrium. The right atrium pumps it into the right ventricle. Blood leaves the right ventricle and passes through the lungs where it picks up oxygen. Newly oxygenated blood returns to the left atrium. The left atrium forces the oxygenated blood into the left ventricle where it is then pumped to the rest of the body.

During systemic circulation, the blood also passes through the kidneys, which filter out much of the waste. Blood also passes through the small intestine and collects in the portal vein, which passes through the liver. The liver filters our remaining waste products and stores glucose from the blood as glycogen.

The Heartbeat

When a doctor uses a stethoscope to hear pulmonary circulation, she listens for the "lub dub." The "lub" is the sound of the tricuspid and mitral valves closing as the two atria pump their contents into the ventricles; the "dub" is the closing of the pulmonary and aortic valves as the two ventricles pump their blood into the pulmonary trunk and aorta.

Arteries

The pulsing of the heart moves blood through the arteries. Arteries continue to divide, becoming smaller and smaller, and eventually turn into capillaries. The most important artery in the body is the aorta, which project from the heart.

An artery, tough on the outside and smooth on the inside, has three layers: an outer layer of tough fibrous tissue known as the adventitia, a smooth muscular middle known as the media, and an inner layer of epithelial cells (the endothelium lining) known as the intima.

The inner layer is very smooth to prevent friction and facilitate blood flow. It is in fact an endocrine gland. Endocrine glands manufacture and secrete hormones locally into the blood stream. These hormones initiate chemical reactions that cause blood vessels, organs, and other body tissues to perform a certain task or tasks. For example, if the blood pressure becomes too high, the endothelium reacts by releasing nitric oxide. Nitric oxide causes the smooth muscle of the media to relax. The endothelium is the largest organ in the body and weighs almost five pounds. If you were to strip it from the arteries and lay it out flat, it would take up about 14,000 square feet.

The elastic muscular wall of the artery (the middle layer) helps the heart pump the blood. It squeezes the artery to make it narrower and relaxes it to make it widen. When the heart beats, the artery expands as it fills with blood. When the heart relaxes, the artery contracts, exerting a force that is strong enough to push the blood along. You can feel your artery expand and contract by taking your pulse.

The arteries deliver the oxygen-rich blood to the capillaries where the actual exchange of oxygen and carbon dioxide occurs. The capillaries then deliver the waste-rich blood to the veins for transport back to the heart and lungs.

Capillaries

Unlike arteries and veins, capillaries are very thin and fragile. They are the smallest of the blood vessels and allow one red blood cell at a time to pass through. Cells are supplied with nutrients and oxygen is diffused through the (one-cell-thick) wall of the capillary. Waste products, including carbon dioxide, are then passed from the cells back through the capillary and enter the bloodstream. The capillaries carrying waste products eventually become larger venules, which then become veins.

Veins

Veins are similar to arteries and have three layers: an outer layer of tissue, muscle in the middle, and a smooth inner layer of epithelial cells. However, the layers of veins are thinner, so they are not as strong as arteries. The most important veins in the body are the vena cavae, which enter the heart.

Veins receive blood from the capillaries after the exchange of oxygen and carbon dioxide has taken place. The veins transport the waste-rich blood back to the lungs and heart. Valves that are located inside the veins prevent the backflow of blood. These valves are necessary to keep blood flowing toward the heart, but they are also necessary to allow blood to flow against the force of gravity. (For example, blood that is returning to the heart from the toes has to be able to flow up the leg.) Vein valves provide necessary footholds, then, for the blood as it climbs its way up.

Blood that flows up to the brain faces the same gravity problem. If the blood is having a hard time climbing up, you will feel lightheaded and possibly even faint. Fainting is your brain's natural request for more oxygen-rich blood. When you faint, your head comes down to the same level as your heart, making it easy for the blood to quickly reach the brain. Efficient solution, really.

Because it lacks oxygen, the waste-rich blood that flows through the veins has a deep red color. And since the walls of the veins are rather thin, this blood is visible through the skin on some parts of the body. Look at your wrist, hands, or ankles. You can probably see your veins carrying your blood back to your heart. Your skin refracts light, though, so that deep red color actually appears a little blue from outside the skin. However, all blood is red.

Blood

Blood makes up about 8% of the body's weight. Adult females have an average of 4.5 liters of blood; adult males, 5.5 liters. Continuous, unobtrusive flow of blood and its constituents is essential to life, as it is the medium by which oxygen and nutrients are delivered to every cell. Here are some other things about blood that you may not know:

Blood protects us from toxins and infectious agents by delivering white blood cells and antibodies to areas of attack.

Blood transports nutrients and waste products to their appropriate sites.

Blood regulates body temperature by transferring heat from muscles to tissues throughout the body, including the capillaries, which help release body heat into the air around us.

Blood regulates body pH by absorbing acids from the interstitial fluid and neutralizing them.

Blood protects the body from harmful toxins and pathogens by way of white-blood-cell reactions.

Blood consists of the following: red cells, which carry oxygen and give blood its color; plasma (the liquid part of blood); white cells, which make up our immune defenses; and platelets, which form clots to protect from bleeding.

Blood plasma is 92% water. Most of plasma is made up of small proteins including albumin. About seven percent of plasma is made up of the protein fibrinogen. The liver makes fibrinogen, which is essential for blood clotting. About 2.5% of plasma is made up of hormones, enzymes, vitamins, electrolytes, and waste material.

Chapter Review

Don't worry. Unlike in your eighth grade health class, there won't really be a test here. But let's hit the highlights one more time.

Blood from the body flows…
by way of the **vena cavae**
to the **right atrium**
through the **tricuspid valve**
to the **right ventricle**
through the **pulmonary valve**
and on to the lungs.

Blood picks up oxygen in the lungs and flows…
through the **pulmonary veins**
to the **left atrium**
through the **mitral valve**
to the **left ventricle**
through the **aortic valve**
and by way of the **aorta**
on to the rest of the body.

Cardiovascular Disease

As you can see, the circulatory system is truly amazing. A healthy heart depends on the circulatory system getting oxygenated blood to the heart by way of the left and right coronary arteries. Unfortunately, for one in three Americans, this system breaks down and results in disease. In the following chapters, we'll explore coronary artery disease, what causes it, how it is traditionally treated, alternative treatments, and ways to prevent it.

Notes

1. E. Horovitz, *Heartbeat: A Complete Guide to Understanding and Preventing Heart Disease* (Los Angeles: Health Trend, 1988).

5

Coronary Artery Disease

THE MOST COMMON TYPE OF HEART DISEASE, coronary artery disease (CAD) affects about 13 million Americans. It causes the loss of oxygen and nutrients to the myocardial (heart) tissue due to poor blood flow through the main artery of the heart.

ATHEROSCLEROSIS

Coronary artery disease (also known as coronary heart disease) is caused by **atherosclerosis,** which is the gradual buildup of plaque on the artery walls. When the walls become fibrous, thick, and calcified, the arterial space narrows, and blood flow is restricted.

The coronary arteries encircle the heart and supply it with oxygen-rich blood. If your coronary arteries become diseased from atherosclerosis, they can't supply enough oxygenated blood to your heart. This insufficient blood supply to the heart is known as cardiac ischemia.

CAD usually develops slowly and silently over decades. Autopsy studies have shown that atherosclerosis may even begin in our early teens. CAD is known as the silent killer, because in 40% of the cases, death is the first symptom!

Those lucky enough to have warning signs might report some of the following.

Angina is often described as a pressure or tightness in the chest and is usually brought on by physical or emotional stress. The pain typically goes away within minutes after stopping the stressful activity. Angina that occurs with exhertion is probably the best indicator of a potential heart attack.

Shortness of breath can develop when CAD leads to congestive heart failure (CHF). Extreme fatigue with exertion, shortness of breath, and swelling in the feet and ankles are the common signs of CHF.

Heart-attack symptoms can occur when one of the arteries that supply the heart with blood becomes completely clogged, either from plaque or a clot. Pain from a heart attack is similar to but more intense than intermittent angina pain. Individuals who have experienced a heart attack describe it as a crushing pain. One person said he felt like an elephant was sitting on his chest. Others describe it as a feeling of intense fullness or a squeezing pain in the center of the chest that lasts for more than a few minutes.

Other reported heart-attack symptoms include pain that radiates to the left shoulder, arm, back, or jaw; increasing episodes of chest pain; prolonged pain in the upper abdomen; shortness of breath; sweating; an impending sense of doom; lightheadedness; fainting; and nausea and vomiting.

Atherosclerosis and Arteriosclerosis

These terms sound very similar. As I explained, atherosclerosis is the buildup of plaque and fatty deposits in the innermost lining of large and medium-sized arteries, particularly the coronary arteries. Over time, these deposits (atheromas) begin to turn to a fibrous plaque that then infiltrates the lining of the arterial wall. These lesions may become hardened in a process known as arteriosclerosis.

Arteriosclerosis is the thickening, stiffening, and calcification of the artery walls. It describes several diseases that involve the cardiovascular system.

It may also occur in the medium and smaller arteries of the body. Then, it is usually referred to as Mönckeberg's sclerosis, which involves the deposition of calcium in the internal layers of the arteries of the lower extremities (legs) and generally leads to an increase in blood pressure.

A third form of the disease is arteriolar sclerosis, which involves both the inner and medial layers of smaller arteries in the arms, legs, eyes, and internal organs. This condition causes decreased blood flow to these tissues, circulatory problems, peripheral vascular disease, and impaired circulation to the eyes and kidneys, causing blindness and kidney failure.

Most individuals with heart disease have a combination of arteriosclerosis (thickening and hardening of the arteries) and atherosclerosis (partial obstruction of the arteries from plaque buildup). This results in arteries that are hard and narrow. Blood has a difficult time circulating through these damaged arteries. Without a sufficient supply of blood and the nutrients it contains, cells begin to die, and organs prematurely age.

Clogged, narrow, diseased arteries cause the heart to work harder and harder in order to supply blood to the trillions of cells contained in the human body. It must work to overcome the resistance caused by the plaque in the arteries. This results in high blood pressure.

In an attempt to pump more blood, the heart increases in size. An enlarged heart requires more nutrients and oxygen and is more vulnerable to the effects of poor circulation associated with coronary artery disease. An enlarged heart may eventually lose its ability to meet the body's demand for blood-carrying oxygen. This then causes the heart itself to become deprived of oxygen and enter a state known as congestive heart failure (CHF).

Inherent Risk Factors

Some risk factors associated with CAD are out of our hands.

Age. Over 83% of people who die of coronary heart disease are 65 or older.

Heredity. Heart disease tends to run in families. African Americans have more severe high blood pressure than do Caucasians and therefore, a higher risk of heart disease. Heart-disease risk is also higher among Mexican Americans, American Indians, native Hawaiians, and some Asian-Americans. This is partly due to higher rates of obesity and diabetes.

Gender. Men have a greater risk of heart attack than women do, and they have attacks earlier in life. Even after menopause, when the death rate from heart disease increases for women, the risk to men is greater.

Baldness. The Department of Medicine at Harvard Medical School and Brigham and Women's Hospital conducted an 11-year study involving over 22,000 male physicians. The study showed that doctors who were bald on top of their heads (as opposed to frontal balding) were more likely to suffer from coronary heart disease, especially when the baldness was combined with other risk factors, such as high blood pressure and high cholesterol.[1]

Treatable Risk Factors

Other risk factors associated with CAD can be treated, modified, or controlled.

Smoking. This one habit increases the risk of dying from a heart attack by 3–5 times. This is also true of chronic exposure to secondhand smoke. One cigarette can increase the heart rate by 20 to 25 beats per minute, and it takes six hours for the circulation to return to normal after one cigarette. Smoking also increases fibrinogen, and increased levels of fibrinogen can cause blood clots. There are 4,000 poisons in tobacco, and some of these toxins deplete vitamin B6, which is essential in reducing high homocysteine levels and so reducing the risk of heart disease. Smoking decreases longevity by an average of 7.5 years. To put it bluntly, 1,000 people die every day from smoking cigarettes.

Physical inactivity. A sedentary lifestyle increases a person's risk of heart disease. But regular physical activity helps prevent heart disease. The more vigorous the activity, the greater the benefits, but even moderate activities help if done regularly and long-term. Exercise can also help control blood cholesterol, type-2 diabetes, obesity, and high blood pressure. The key is consistent, daily (or every other day) activities that get your heart rate up for a continuous period of time. Brisk walking, light jogging, swimming, or other aerobic activities for 30–60 minutes a day can provide substantial benefits.

Obesity. People with excess body fat—especially if concentrated around the waist (such as with a pear-shaped body)—are more likely to develop heart disease and stroke, even if they have no other risk factors. It increases the risk of type-2 diabetes, raises blood pressure, and increases blood cholesterol levels and triglycerides while lowering HDL (good) cholesterol and increasing the body's resistance to inslulin.

Insulin is a hormone responsible for delivering glucose (blood sugar) into the cells where it is used as fuel. Excess fat cells can block insulin receptors and increase the risk of sugar being deposited in the *arteries* instead. This can start a chain reaction that results in arteriosclerosis and heart disease.

Increased fat cells also cause the heart and cardiovascular system to work harder. It is estimated that it takes one mile of capillaries to supply each pound of fat. What if you are 10 to 20 pounds overweight? This translates into 10 to 20 extra miles of capillaries that must be serviced by the heart.

Losing just 10 pounds of weight results in an average decreased systolic pressure of seven points and a drop of five points in diastolic pressure. A one-point drop in diastolic pressure results in a 3% decreased risk of heart disease and a 7% decreased risk of stroke.[2]

Conversely, a weight gain of 10% can increase systolic blood pressure by 6.5 points. Total cholesterol typically increases 12 points for every 10% increase in weight gain.[3]

Diabetes. Diabetes (both type-1 and type-2) seriously increases your risk of developing cardiovascular disease. About 3/4 of people with diabetes die of some form of heart or blood vessel disease.

Stress. Individual response to stress may be a contributing factor in the progression of CAD. Chronic stress increases the release of hormones associated with producing inflammation and atherosclerotic damage.

Alcohol overuse. Drinking too much alcohol can raise blood pressure, cause heart failure, and lead to stroke. It can contribute to high triglycerides, cancer and other diseases, and irregular heartbeats. However, for those of you who like to have a glass of wine or a beer once and awhile, read on. The risk of heart disease in people who drink moderate amounts of alcohol (an average of one drink for women or two drinks for men per day) is lower than in nondrinkers. One drink is defined as 1.5 oz. 80-proof spirits (such as bourbon, Scotch, vodka, or gin), 1 oz. 100-proof spirits, 4 oz. wine, or 12 oz. beer.

Hypothyroidism. An underactive thyroid increases the risk of arteriosclerosis because it raises cholesterol and triglycerides.[4]

Hypertension. High blood pressure (hypertension) increases the heart's workload, causing it to thicken and become stiffer. It also increases your risk of stroke, heart attack, kidney failure, and congestive heart failure. When high blood pressure exists with obesity, smoking, high blood-cholesterol levels, or diabetes, the risk of heart attack or stroke increases several times. High blood pressure is epidemic in America. In the next chapter, I will explain hypertension in detail.

The Strange Significance of Earlobe Creases

At least 30 different studies have shown that a diagonal crease in the earlobe was a sign of increased risk for heart attack. The presence of a unilateral earlobe crease was associated with a 33% increase in the risk of heart attack and 77% if both earlobes were creased.

Chronic circulatory problems cause the blood vessels in the earlobe to collapse. This then creates a crease in the earlobe. A diagonal earlobe crease is a better indicator of sudden death from heart attack than are age, smoking, weight, high cholesterol, or a sedentary lifestyle. For some reason, a creased earlobe does not increase the risk of heart attack in Asians and Native Americans.[5,6]

Notes

1. P.A. Lotufo et al., "Male Pattern Baldness and Coronary Heart Disease: the Physicians' Health Study," *Archives of Internal Medicine* 160(2) (2000): 165–71.
2. Mark Houston, *What Your Doctor May Not Tell You About Hypertension* (New York: Time Warner, 2003).
3. ibid.
4. B.U. Althaus et al., "LDL/HDL Changes in Subclinical Hypothroidism: Possible Rick Factors for Coronary Heart Disease," *British Medical Journal* 290 (1985): 1555–1561.
5. W.J. Elliott, "Ear Lobe Crease and Coronary Artery Disease: 1,000 Patients and Review of the Literature," *American Journal of Medicine* 75(6) (1983): 1024–32.
6. W.J. Elliott and L.H. Powell, "Diagonal Earlobe Creases and Prognosis in Patients with Suspected Coronary Artery Disease," *American Journal of Medicine* 100(2) (February 1996): 205–11.

6

Bringing Down Your Blood Pressure

OVER 50 MILLION AMERICANS suffer from hypertension, also known as high blood pressure. That's one out of every four adults. In 2002, nearly 43,000 Americans died from hypertension, and another 227,000 died from causes related to it.[1]

WHAT IS BLOOD PRESSURE?

Blood is carried from the heart to all parts of your body in vessels called arteries, and blood pressure is a measurement of the force of your blood pushing against the walls of your arteries. Each time the heart beats (about 60–70 times a minute when we're at rest), it is pumping out blood. It is at this moment that your blood pressure is at its highest. The measure of pressure on your arteries while your heart pumps is called systolic pressure. When the heart is at rest, between beats, your blood pressure falls. This is your diastolic pressure.

Blood pressure changes during the day. It is lowest as you sleep and rises when you get up. It also can rise when you are excited, nervous, or active.

Blood pressure is measured by using a sphygmomanometer (blood-pressure cuff) and a stethoscope. The cuff is inflated around the brachial artery in your upper arm, and your doctor or nurse listens to the tapping sounds caused by your blood within your arteries. The systolic pressure is measured first, while the cuff is inflated. The diastolic pressure is measured after the cuff begins to deflate. Your blood pressure measurement will then be reported as a fraction, with the systolic number listed above the diastolic. For instance, normal blood pressure is around 120/80.

Hypertension is diagnosed when the systolic pressure is above 140 or the diastolic pressure is above 90. Blood pressure that is between normal and hypertensive is considered **pre-hypertensive.**

Stage-1 hypertension occurs when the systolic pressure is 140–159 or the diastolic pressure is 90–99. **Stage-2 hypertension** occurs when the systolic pressure is above 160 or the diastolic pressure is above 100.

Why is Hypertension Dangerous?

Our arteries and veins are like garden hoses that carry our blood throughout our bodies in order to nurture our garden of living cells. Recall from chapter 4, though, that unlike rubber hoses, our blood vessels are living flesh. Their layers of functioning tissue act as an organ to perform vital bodily functions. The middle layer of smooth muscle tightens and relaxes, causing the blood vessel to become narrower or wider. This is one way that the arterial system works to control blood pressure and blood volume—contracting and relaxing with the cadence of your beating heart.

But perhaps the most complex layer of the artery is the endothelium, the inner layer, which is actually an endocrine gland. The increased force caused by excess blood pressure can damage this fragile endothelial lining. Damage to the endothelium interferes with its ability to secrete hormones and other substances that help control blood pressure, the stickiness of the blood, the growth of the blood vessel wall, and other essential blood functions. Damage to the blood-vessel wall can further cause atherosclerosis, or hardening of the arteries. All these effects can lead to some serious problems.

The heart can grow in size in order to compensate. This can lead to congestive heart failure as explained earlier in the book.

Small bulges (aneurysms) can form in the blood vessels.

Common locations for aneurysms are the aorta (the main artery from the heart), the artery leading to the spleen, and arteries in the brain, legs, and intestines.

Blood vessels in the kidney can narrow. This may cause kidney failure.

Arteries throughout the body can become atherosclerotic faster, especially in the heart, brain, kidneys, and legs. This can lead to a heart attack, a stroke, or kidney failure.

Blood vessels in the eyes can burst or bleed, which may cause vision changes and even blindness.

Heart attack and stroke risk increases. Individuals with stage-1 hypertension suffer a 31% greater risk of heart attack, almost twice the risk of stroke, and a 43% higher death rate than those with normal blood pressure.[2]

What Causes Hypertension?

Essential hypertension is high blood pressure that has no definitive cause. This is the case for 95% of those with hypertension.

Secondary hypertension is high blood pressure due to another condition, such as kidney disease, diabetes, prescription medications, allergic reactions, and chemical sensitivities.

How is it Treated?

Typically, hypertension is treated with drugs, including diuretics (water pills), calcium channel blockers, beta-blockers, ACE inhibitors, and specific vasodilators. You can read more about these in chapter 2.

For many people, taking a pill seems at first like a simple solution. But you now know that every prescription blood-pressure drug has potential side effects. In the case of calcium channel blockers, one side effect is a possible heart attack or stroke! Beta-blockers, diuretics, and ACE inhibitor drugs are also associated with several serious side effects that are often more dangerous than the hypertension itself. When these side effects are treated with more prescription drugs that then create more symptoms, the result is an insane cycle of suffering. There is a better way.

High blood pressure is not to be taken lightly. However, it never ceases to amaze me the number of men and women who are placed on potentially life-threatening medications for minimally elevated blood pressure. Especially since most of these individuals have never been educated on natural ways to reduce their hypertension. Diet modification and exercise alone will often be all that is needed.

The author of *Worst Pills, Best Pills* elaborate on studies that demonstrate that most individuals with high blood pressure can and should use diet, exercise, and weight reduction to treat their condition instead. "The results of this study and decades of extensive research now make it possible to speak in terms of preventing high blood pressure rather than treating it with drugs, which is defensive, mainly reactive, time-consuming, associated with adverse drugs effects, costly, only partially successful, endless, and is not a cure."[3]

I'm going to introduce you to an excellent alternative to dangerous hypertension drugs: nutritional supplements (along with a healthy diet and lifestyle). It's not as easy as popping a pill, but for many people, it's a whole lot healthier and safer. Studies show that for 2/3 of individuals taking high-blood-pressure medication, diet therapy alone will result in normal blood pressure.[4]

If you try my plan and still can't get your blood pressure down naturally, then by all means, consult your medical doctor and see which prescription medication is right for you. But please remember the less is best. And which medication you take matters, too. The ACE and angiotensin drugs appear to have the least harmful side effects. And if you are taking prescription medications, you can still take your nutritional supplements. However, you'll then need to monitor your blood pressure on a daily basis, since adding nutritional supplements to your prescription medications can cause drastic blood pressure reductions.

If you're already on drugs for hypertension, *do not stop taking your prescription medications without first consulting the doctor who prescribed them.* Many of the drugs used to treat high blood pressure and heart disease need to be slowly discontinued over a period of time. Trying to discontinue certain medications too quickly may cause a host of unwanted withdrawal symptoms.

Still, it's not impossible to get off of your high-blood-pressure medication (with your doctor's help). Too often, patients falsely assume they will have to stay on them for the rest of their lives. There is no truth to this. In fact, a recent editorial in the *British Medical Journal* pointed out that the "treatment of hypertension is part of preventive medicine and like all preventive strategies, its progress should be regularly reviewed by whoever initiates it.... Patients should no longer be told that treatment is necessary for life: the possibility of reducing or stopping treatment should be mentioned at the outset."[5]

Reducing Hypertension Naturally

There are several steps you can take to naturally and safely lower your blood pressure.

Start monitoring your own blood pressure. Checking it once in a while at the doctor's office or when you have time at the pharmacy isn't going to help you much. You should be able to buy an automated, battery-powered blood sphygmomanometer at your local pharmacy. Check yourself daily at least. There's no reason to wonder if your treatment is working.

Limit your salt intake to no more than 2,000 mg. a day. It is estimated that up to 60% of hypertensive patients are salt-sensitive. You can easily reduce your salt by eliminating processed foods, which account for about 75% of our sodium intake. Studies have demonstrated that salt-restricted diets can reduce systolic pressure by 11.5 and diastolic pressure by 6.8. Another study involving individuals taking hypertensive medications showed that a third of those with hypertension could discontinue their medications by restricting their salt intake to less than 1,800 milligrams per day and losing 10 pounds.[6]

Americans consume 6–10 grams of salt per day. We actually only need about half a gram (500 mg.) daily. A daily salt intake of 1,500 to 2,000 mg. a day is certainly doable and yet low enough to help reduce high blood pressure.

Reducing your salt intake can be complicated at first. Many common foods contain large amounts of salt. Be sure to read the label and look for low-salt versions of these products: baking powder, baking soda, bouillon, buttermilk, processed cheese, cottage cheese, crackers, pretzels, potato chips, corn chips, ketchup, popcorn, processed nuts, olives, canned or processed meats, monosodium glutamate (listed as MSG), pickles, salad dressings, prepackaged soups, and many sauces such as soy sauce, teriyaki sauce, and steak sauce.

Start a daily exercise program. Simply walking 30–60 minutes a day can yield tremendous health benefits. Start slowly, and increase your exercise time gradually over a period of weeks.

If you're overweight, set a goal to lose those unwanted pounds. Remember, losing just 10 pounds of weight results in an average of 7 points lower systolic pressure and 5 points lower diastolic. Work with your doctor on this, and celebrate each milestone.

Increase your fiber intake. Studies show that by increasing fiber-rich fruits, vegetables, and whole grains—or by taking fiber supplements—a person can, on average, drop his systolic number by 10 and his diastolic number by 5.[7] Good sources of fiber include fruits, vegetables, nuts, and whole grains.

Get your fish oil. Eat a minimum of two deep-sea, cold-water fish a week (such as salmon), or take 2,000–3,000 mg. of fish oil a day. Fish oil reduces blood pressure, inflammation, fibrinogen, irregular heartbeats (arrhythmia), atherosclerosis, triglycerides, and platelet aggregation.[8] The *New England Journal of Medicine* reported that in individuals who consumed 15 g. of fish oil a day, blood pressure dropped significantly. Typically, 4–7 g. of fish oil are needed for a 1.6–2.9 drop in blood pressure. If the dose is increased to 15 g., blood pressure drops 5.8–8.1.[9] Individuals who lose weight and take fish oil supplements may reduce their systolic blood pressure by 13 points and their diastolic by 9 points.[10]

Simply eating 2–3 servings of deep-sea, cold-water fish a week or taking 2–3 g. of fish-oil supplements daily are great ways to decrease your overall risk of hypertension and CAD.

Get plenty of antioxidants, found in most fruits and vegetables. Several studies have shown that increasing the daily intake of antioxidant-rich foods helps reduce high blood pressure. One antioxidant, lycopene, has the ability to lower both systolic and diastolic pressure by up to 10 points.[11] Lycopene is found in tomatoes, guavas, pink grapefruit, watermelon, papayas, red peppers, and strawberries. Other antioxidant-rich foods include apples, pears, oranges, blueberries, squash, green beans, spinach, broccoli, baby lettuces, and other fruits and vegetables.

Supplement with 100–200 mg. of CoQ10 a day. Anyone suspected to be in any stage of CAD should be taking CoQ10, as it significantly improves diastolic and systolic pressure in essential hypertension. In one study, more than half of the patients receiving 225 mg. of CoQ10 a day were able to terminate the use of 1–3 antihypertensive medications. Those taking 100–225 mg. of CoQ10 a day reduced their systolic blood pressure by an average of 15 points and diastolic pressure by 10 points.[12] You can read all about this amazing enzyme in chapter 9.

Take a quality multivitamin every day. It should be based on the optimal daily allowance (ODA) of nutrients, not the "recommended" daily allowance (RDA). Look for a multivitamin containing at least of 500 mg. of magnesium; plenty of the vitamins C, E, D, and the Bs; and calcium, potassium, and zinc. Here's why.

Individuals who consume a minimum of 800 mg. of calcium per day are 23% less likely to develop high blood pressure.[13] Potassium helps to balance the effects of sodium (salt). That's because they are designed to work together to balance blood pressure. Potassium helps relax blood vessels, and sodium does just the opposite. By increasing potassium and reducing salt, a person can see some very positive changes in blood pressure. Several double-blind, placebo-controlled studies have shown that vitamin C helps reduce elevated blood pressure by up to 10 points.[14] In fact, combining vitamin C with vitamin E inhibits plaque growth. And vitamin E taken in doses of 400–1,000 IUs daily has been shown to reduce oxidized cholesterol (one source of cardiovascular disease), lower blood pressure, and boost nitric oxide levels. It also reduces the formation of blood clots and plaque. Combining calcium with vitamin D helps reduce blood pressure by an average of 9 points.[15]

Supplement with niacin (vitamin B3). It has been used as an antilipid medicine for decades and is the only vitamin supplement listed as a potential drug for treating high cholesterol (Niaspan). Of course, prescription niacin costs over $180 for a one-month supply, while over-the-counter niacin costs around $20 a month.

Niacin, when taken in high doses, often lowers systolic and diastolic blood pressure. However, it is associated with a histamine release that causes a flushing sensation. This flushing can be quite uncomfortable. Timed-release niacin offers a way around this reaction, but for some sensitive individuals, even the timed-release niacin may cause flushing. And there are reports that timed-release niacin can cause elevated liver enzymes. It may be best to use a special form of niacin called no-flush niacin (inositol hexaniacinate or IHN). It appears to be safe and free of side effects at doses up to four grams a day.[16] I routinely use IHN and find it to be a safe and effective way to lower high blood pressure.

Niacin is also more effective than statin drugs at lowering fibrinogen (a protein associated with inflammation), raising HDL cholesterol, and lowering LDL cholesterol. Niacin has been shown to raise HDL by 29% while lowering triglycerides (fats) by 28% and total cholesterol by 16%.[17]

The recommended dose of timed-release or no-flush niacin is 400–500 mg. a day for 3–4 days. You can then increase to 500 mg. twice a day for 3–4 days. Once again, you can increase the dose by 400–500 mg. for another 3–4 days. Keep adding 400–500 mg. in divided doses until you reach 2,000–3,000 mg. a day, or until your blood pressure begins to drop. (Remember, you're checking it daily at least.)

When your blood pressure does begin to drop, continue to monitor it and, after several days, try to reduce your daily dose of niacin. *If you are taking prescription drugs along with IHN, make sure you check your blood pressure 2–3 times a day, every day.* IHN is potent. Don't let your blood pressure drop below 100/80, or you may start to feel lousy.

Additional Supplements That Can Help a Lot

Consider these supplements your secret weapons in the battle against hypertension.

Ameal peptide is a natural substance consisting of two peptides derived from fermented milk. Fourteen double-blind, placebo-controlled clinical studies have shown that ameal peptide lowers high blood pressure.[18] It acts like an angiotensin drug or ACE drug but without the side effects. Ameal peptide inhibits angiotensin I changing to angiotensin II, allowing blood vessels to remain unconstricted and maintain normal blood pressure. It's safe to use with other medications. *Caution: If you add ameal peptide to your current blood-pressure medications, you must monitor your blood pressure several times a day to avoid dropping too low.* If your blood pressure does drop below 100/80, reduce your ameal peptide. Then talk to your doctor about reducing your current blood-pressure medication. Continue to work with your doctor to adjust your prescriptions as your blood pressure decreases.

Over 300 million doses of ameal peptide have been sold worldwide with no reported side effects. People with lactose intolerance or milk-protein allergies can still safely use ameal peptide.

Nattokinase is a potent fibrinolytic (anticlotting) enzyme extracted from natto, a traditional Japanese fermented, cheese-like food. Natto has been used for over 1,000 years to treat heart and vascular disorders. Nattokinase enhances the body's ability to prevent and reverse blood clots, without the potential side effects of prescription anticlotting medications like Cumadin and Plavix.

As if 1,000 years of results isn't enough to convince us, nattokinase has undergone numerous scientific studies. Research has shown that nattokinase supports the body's ability to break up and dissolve the unhealthy coagulation of blood. In fact, it has been shown to have four times greater fibrinolytic activity than plasmin—the body's primary anticlotting enzyme.[19]

Animal trials have shown that nattokinase is able to dissolve a blood clot in the carotid artery, increasing blood flow by 62%—while blood flow of those treated with traditional drugs improved less than 16%.[20] Clinical studies involving human volunteers with high blood pressure showed a decrease in systolic pressure (from 173 to 154) and diastolic pressure dropping by an average of 10 points.[21,22]

L-arginine is an amino acid that acts as a potent vasodilator, because it increases the production of nitric oxide (ever hear of nitroglycerin tablets?), which relaxes the muscles of the blood vessels and so lowers blood pressure. (By the way, the "L" just refers to the form of the arginine.) L-arginine keeps platelets from sticking to the blood vessel wall and in this way helps to prevent blood clots, heart attack, and stroke. It slows plaque growth and even suppresses arteriosclerosis.[23] Arginine can reduce high blood pressure when taken on its own in high doses (7 g. a day). However, if you use a combination of strategies as I'm outlining here, you'll not need to take a high dose. A little will go a long way.

A New Way to Pop Pills for Hypertension

Along with limiting your salt, achieving a healthy weight, and eating plenty of fiber, antioxidants, and fish oils, you will have a few pills to "pop" on my plan.

- Take your CoQ10.
- Take your high-quality multivitamin daily.
- Take you niacin as described above (be sure to account for any niacin already in your multivitamin).
- If still needed, supplement with ameal peptide, nattokinase, and arginine. I recommend to my hypertension patients a special formula called Cardio-Stolix. It's produced by Douglas Laboratories and contains ameal peptide, nattokinase, and L-arginine (as well as the natural herb hawthorne, magnesium, and other helpful nutrients). It's available only to physicians, though, so ask your doctor about ordering it for you from Douglas Laboratories. Or you can order my BP Support Formula, which is the same formulation as Cardio-Stolix. See the appendix for ordering information.

Notes

1. Mark Houston, *What Your Doctor May Not Tell You About Hypertension* (New York: Time Warner, 2003).
2. ibid.
3. Sidney M. Wolfe, *Worst Pills Best Pills: A Consumer's Guide to Preventing Drug-Induced Death* (New York: Pocket, 1999), 46.
4. R. Stamler et al., "Nutritional Therapy for High Blood Pressure," *Journal of the American Medical Association* 257(11) (1987): 1484–91.
5. R. Burton, "Withdrawing Antihypertensive Treatment: Hypertension May Settle with Time," *British Medical Journal* 303 (1991): 324–5.
6. Mark Houston, *What Your Doctor May Not Tell You About Hypertension* (New York: Time Warner, 2003).
7. P. Sclamowitz et al., "Treatment of Mild to Moderate Hypertension with Dietary Fibre," *Lancet* 8559 (1987): 622–3.
8. Life Extension Media, *Disease and Prevention*, 4th ed. (Hollywood: Life Extension Media, 2003): 443–5.
9. H.R. Knapp and G.A. Fitzgerald, "The Antihypertensive Effects of Fish Oil: A Controlled Study of Polyunsaturated Fatty Acid Supplements in Essential Hypertension," *New England Journal of Medicine* 320 (1989): 1037–1043.
10. M. Morris, F. Sacks, and B. Rosner, "Does Fish Oil Lower Blood Pressure? A Meta-analysis of Controlled Trials," *Circulation* 88 (1993): 523–33.
11. E. Paran and Y.N. Englehard, "Effects of Lycopene, an Oral Natural Antioxidant, on Blood Pressure," *Journal of Hypertension* 19 (2001): 574.
12. P. Langjoen, R. Willis, and K. Folkers, "Treatment of Essential Hypertension with Coenzyme Q10," *Molecular Aspects of Medicine* 15 (1994): S265–72.
13. Mark Houston, *What Your Doctor May Not Tell You About Hypertension* (New York: Time Warner, 2003).
14. D.L. Trout, "Vitamin C and Cardiovascular Risk Factors," *American Journal of Clinical Nutrition* 53 (1991): 322–5.
15. M. Pfeifer et al., "Effects of Short Term Vitamin D (3) and Calcium Supplementation on Blood Pressure and Parathyroid Hormone Levels in Elderly Women," *Journal of Clinical Endocrinology and Metabolism* 86 (2001): 1633–7.
16. A.L. Welsh and M. Ede, "Inositol Hexanicotinate for Improved Nicotinic Acid Therapy," *International Record of Medicine* 174 (1961): 9–15.
17. M.B. Elam, "Effect of Niacin on Lipid and Lipoprotein Levels and Glycemic Control in Patients with Diabetes and Peripheral Arterial Disease," *Journal of the American Medical Association* 248 (2000): 1263–70.
18. Medical News Today, "Blood Pressure Lowered By Calpis' Ameal Peptide In 2 Placebo-Controlled Trials" (2008), www.medicalnewstoday.com/articles/107888.php.
19. Y. Suzuki et al., "Dietary Supplementation with Fermented Soybeans Suppresses Intimal Thickening," *Nutrition* 19(3) (March 2003): 261–4.

20. M. Fujita et al., "Thrombolytic Effect of Nattokinase on Chemically Induced Thrombosis Model in Rat," *Biological and Pharmaceutical Bulletin* 18(10) (October 1995): 1387–91.
21. H. Sumi et al., "Enhancement of the Fibrinolytic Activity in Plasma by Oral Administration of Nattokinase," *Acta Haematologica 84 (1990): 139–43.*
22. Smart Publications Authors, "Nattokinase—The Natural Blood Thinner," web article (accessed August 2008), www.smart-publications.com/heart_attacks/nattokinase_naturalbloodthinner.php.
23. Sherry Rogers, *The High Blood Pressure Hoax* (Syracuse: Prestige, 2008): 29–30.

7

Cholesterol Myths and Facts

I HAVE HAD TO RELEARN EVERYTHING I had ever learned about cholesterol. And I'm going to do my best to teach it to you here. This is not an easy concept to explain. Lipoproteins, low-density lipids, very low-density lipids, triglycerides, and other terms having to do with cholesterol do not generally come up at cocktail parties. So I've worked to make this chapter not only as honest as possible but easy to understand, too.

Many years ago, I was an advocate of a strict low-fat, low-cholesterol diet. I even practiced the Pritikin diet, one of the low-fat diets so popular several years ago, myself. (This was "B.S.B." [before South Beach], but I digress.)

Nathanial Pritikin was a layman who set out to lower his cholesterol levels to rock bottom numbers after he found out he had advanced CAD. His zealous promotion of his low-fat lifestyle won over many converts, and he became quite famous. Pritikin was able to beat heart disease, but when faced with leukemia, he elected to commit suicide. His tragic situation may have even been caused by the very thing that Pritikin promoted: his low-fat diet.

Unbelievable? A low-fat diet can cause cancer and even suicide? As a reformed low-fat, low-cholesterol advocate myself, I can sympathize with your shock and dismay. However, since you purchased this book, you already know from the title that I don't intend to pull any punches. In fact, I'm going to attempt to dispel all the medical myths that claim cholesterol and fat are evil villains that should be purged from our diets. My task isn't easy, because this cholesterol myth has taken a real foothold in the public's mind.

What is Cholesterol?

Cholesterol is a soft, waxy, fat-like substance manufactured in your liver. It's found in all animals. (Chemically, cholesterol is really an alcohol, but it's a lot like a fat, and so we'll treat it like one here.) Since cholesterol is not soluble in blood (or water), the liver coats it with a protein shell so that it can be transported to and from the cells. These carrier shells are called lipoproteins.

High-density lipoproteins (HDLs) carry cholesterol away from the arteries and back to the liver, where most of it is passed from the body. About 1/3 of blood cholesterol is carried by these HDLs.

Low-density lipoproteins (LDLs) and very-low-density lipoproteins (VLDLs) deliver cholesterol to the cells of the body, where it sticks around. Cells that need cholesterol have receptor sites for it. It is at these receptor sites that the LDL attaches to the cell. Then the cholesterol within the LDL is pulled inside the cell, where it is used for a variety of functions.

Not all the body's cells can accept cholesterol, however. Those that don't need or use it aren't equipped to accept it. That means that no matter how much cholesterol is circulating in the bloodstream, no cell is going to become overfilled with cholesterol. If a cell doesn't use it or doesn't need any more, it will just keep circulating.

So one thing should be clear by now: lipoproteins are *not* cholesterol. They are carrier molecules that transport cholesterol. We refer to "LDL cholesterol" as the cholesterol carried by the LDLs and "HDL cholesterol" as that carried by the HDLs.

Give Cholesterol a Chance

When you say the word *cholesterol* today, people cringe. It has become synonymous with sludge. For goodness's sake…it's not poison. It's a nutrient!

Cholesterol and fats are the very building blocks that make up each and every cell. Cholesterol is an important fat that helps keep cell membranes permeable. This permeability allows good nutrients to get in and toxic waste products to get out of the cell. Cholesterol is the precursor to vitamin D, which is necessary for numerous biochemical processes, including mineral metabolism. Cholesterol makes the bile salts required for the digestion of fat. That's why those with low cholesterol levels often suffer from bloating, gas, and indigestion. These bile salts also allow us to digest fat-soluble vitamins, including vitamins A, K, D, and E. A deficiency in any one of these vitamins can cause a host of health problems, including depression, bone loss, poor immune function, leaky-gut syndrome, chronic pain, and cancer.

Cholesterol is used by the body to repair and patch damaged cellular membranes; scar tissue contains a lot of cholesterol. This is one of the reasons cholesterol is seen in arterial plaques. When an arterial cell is damaged from free radicals, infection, or other inflammatory processes, cholesterol is dispatched to patch the diseased tissue. Cholesterol is definitely not the cause of atherosclerosis. Rather, it helps us survive in spite of atherosclerosis, which is a by-product of the damage-and-repair cycle.

Over 8% of the brain's solid matter is made up of cholesterol. Fats in general make up 70% of the brain. Fat insulates the brain cells, allowing neurotransmitters (hormones including serotonin, dopamine, and epinephrine) to communicate with one another. Fat and cholesterol is essential for proper brain function and normalized moods. That's why low cholesterol has been linked to certain mood disorders, including depression and anxiety.

Cholesterol is also essential in maintaining proper hormone production. Testosterone, dehydroepiandrosterone (DHEA), progesterone, estradiol, and cortisol are all made from cholesterol.

Because cholesterol is essential to our very survival, the body manufactures 800–1,500 mg. of it each day.

Five Cholesterol Myths

Myth 1: High cholesterol causes CAD. Nope. But you say, "I just don't believe this. Doesn't everyone believe that cholesterol causes atherosclerosis or clogging of the arteries?" Not by a long shot. In fact, some of the brightest scientists, PhDs, and medical doctors do not believe cholesterol causes atherosclerosis. Even I have finally come around and realized what these brave medical mavericks have staunchly claimed: cholesterol levels have nothing to do with increasing the risk of heart disease.

Actually, low cholesterol levels may cause heart attacks, but not high cholesterol. Read what the Journal of Cardiology had to say on this matter: "Low cholesterol increases the risk of a heart attack."[1] And it actually doubles the risk of death. That's because when there's not enough cholesterol in the body, calcium channel pumps don't work properly. This can cause irregular heartbeat, chest pain, high blood pressure, and congestive heart failure.[2,3]

Study after study has shown that there is no relationship between blood cholesterol levels and the degree of atherosclerosis in the vessels. For instance, research conducted at the Department of Forensic Medicine of New York University in 1936 found absolutely no correlation between the amount of cholesterol in the blood and the degree of atherosclerosis.[4] Almost 30 years later, researchers sampled the blood of over 800 war veterans and came to the conclusion that there was no connection between their degree of atherosclerosis and their blood-cholesterol levels. Those with low cholesterol levels had as much plaque as those with high cholesterol levels. And those who had low cholesterol were just as atherosclerotic when they died as those who had high cholesterol. In other words, their cholesterol could not have been causing their atherosclerosis.[5] Another prestigious medical journal, *the Lancet,* reported in 1994 that most individuals with coronary artery disease have normal cholesterol levels.[6]

So why do so many physicians still believe that cholesterol levels are linked to CAD? A big culprit is the Framingham study. This study, begun in 1948 and conducted over a 14-year period, measured the cholesterol levels of 2,282 men and 2,845 women. The study's authors found that the higher a person's cholesterol level, the greater his risk of heart disease. Since then, the Framingham study has been held as the gold standard for proving the theory that high cholesterol levels cause CAD. However, there is a growing list of medical scientists who are now questioning the methods and results of this and other studies with similar "results." One follow-up to the Framingham study focuses on the apparently overlooked fact that as cholesterol levels dropped in study participants, the risk of death increased. To cite the Framingham authors, "For each 1 mg/dl drop of cholesterol there was an 11% increase in coronary and total mortality."[7]

It's not that this clarifying research doesn't show up in the medical journals. It does. It's just often ignored. Perhaps the pharmaceutical companies' aggressive ad campaigns that fill both medical journals and the media at large have something to do with it. They have quite a vested interest in perpetuating the cholesterol myth, considering that cholesterol-lowering statin medications account for 6.5% of all drug sales in the United States, or 25 billion dollars. That's $25,000,000,000.00! Lipitor *alone* accounts for $10 billion dollars of this total.

Other studies have shown that cholesterol numbers, especially total cholesterol levels, may not be as important as we have been led to believe. It appears that total cholesterol is not a very reliable marker for predicting the risk of a heart attack in men above age 65.[8] In a 30-year follow-up of the Framingham population, for instance, high cholesterol was not predictive at all after the age of 47, and those whose cholesterol went down had the highest risk of heart attack.[9]

Yes, you read that right—straight from a medical journal. Anyone over the age of 47 who is taking cholesterol-lowering drugs should read chapter 8 and seriously reconsider their choices.

Myth 2: LDL cholesterol is "bad" cholesterol. Why would it be bad? It provides an essential bodily function. Doctors continue to rail against the dangers of high LDL levels. However, the research clearly shows that *it doesn't really matter* whether or not LDL is elevated. Half of those with demonstrative heart disease have normal LDL levels. For example, for the 28,000 participants in the Women's Health Study, 46% of first-time cardiovascular events (heart attacks, strokes, etc.) occurred in individuals with normal LDL levels.[10]

Only when LDL cholesterol becomes *oxidized* from free-radical proliferation does it become harmful. Naturally, oxidized LDL is a far better predictor of arteriosclerosis and full-blow cardiovascular disease than are LDL levels alone. Since oxidized LDL is what's dangerous, free-radical damage is what causes LDL to oxidize, and antioxidants prevent free-radical damage, it's your *antioxidant* level that's important.

In animal studies, antioxidants have been shown to impair oxidized LDL and reverse arteriosclerosis despite cholesterol amount levels.[11] Studies in humans have shown that oxidized LDL levels substantially increase the risk of heart attack and stroke, no matter what the person's cholesterol level.[12]

This information is nothing new—conveniently ignored, but not new. Researchers have reported on the dangers of oxidized LDL levels for over a decade. In 1997, Swedish researchers evaluated two seemingly similar groups of men—one from Vilnius, Lithuania, and one from Linkoping, Sweden. There were few if any traditional risk factors between the two groups. However, the Lithuanian group had a four-fold higher death rate from cardiovascular disease then their Swedish counterparts. Interestingly enough, the Lithuanians had the lower LDL levels! But as you may have guessed, the Lithuanians had significantly higher concentrations of *oxidized* LDL. They also had decreased levels of antioxidant nutrients including beta carotene, lycopene, and vitamin E.[13] Sounds like keeping your diet full of antioxidant-rich foods might just be more important than eating less cholesterol. You think? Which brings us to our next myth....

Myth 3: Eating a low-cholesterol diet reduces blood cholesterol levels. Low-cholesterol diets are *rarely* successful in reducing blood cholesterol. That's because reducing dietary cholesterol only triggers the body to make more.

Humans only get 15% of their daily cholesterol from eating animal products, dairy, meats, fish, and shellfish. The majority of cholesterol is produced by the human body. And we have a self-regulating cholesterol meter that monitors our daily cholesterol production. If you reduce the amount of cholesterol you ingest, your body will simply adjust by manufacturing more. Only a small percentage of people find they can actually reduce their cholesterol levels with low-fat dieting alone.

Myth 4: Eating a high-cholesterol diet increases blood cholesterol levels. You ask, "What about eating filet mignon, eggs, butter, and other delicious foods high in cholesterol? Will this raise my cholesterol levels?" I know that for those of you on the American Heart Association's low-fat, low-cholesterol diet, this will be difficult to swallow (pun intended). But the answer is no. In fact, you'll actually lower your cholesterol levels. (I will explain this more thoroughly in chapter 12, but for now, let me share this basic biochemical fact: Dietary fat does not turn into fat. Unused carbohydrates turn into fat.)

By 1998, there were a total of 30 different studies—involving more than 150,000 people—that looked at the relationship of dietary fat to the risk of heart disease. These studies showed there was *no* difference in the risk of CAD in those who ate animal fats and those who did not.[14]

The fat intake for many countries has increased over the years, but the increase in fat intake does not appear to be related to any particular change in number of CAD cases. For example, take a look at Greece, the birthplace of the Mediterranean Diet. Comparing the amount of fat intake during the years 1961–1963 to that of 1983–1985 shows that the people of Greece increased their consumption of saturated fats by 65%. Yet their incidence of heart disease only increased by 13%. To quote Ancel Keys of Mediterranean Diet fame, from a paper in 1956, "In the adult man the serum cholesterol level is essentially independent of the cholesterol intake over the whole range of human diets." This means that it didn't matter what kind of diet they ate: high cholesterol, low cholesterol, low fat, or high fat. More recently, Dr. Keys had this to say about the connection between cholesterol in the diet and cholesterol in the blood: "There's no connection whatsoever between cholesterol in food and cholesterol in blood. And we've known that all along. Cholesterol in the diet doesn't matter at all unless you happen to be a chicken or a rabbit."[15,16] Dr. Keys says it so eloquently.

In 1976, a study was performed by a team of researchers from the University of Michigan headed by Dr. Allen Nichols. Experienced dieticians meticulously screened over 2,000 individuals and analyzed over 3,000 American food items to make their scientific calculations. There was no relation between the amount of saturated fat in the diet and blood cholesterol.[17]

For those who need more proof that eating fatty, cholesterol-laden foods does not cause an increase in cholesterol levels—or it you just love to read through technical reports—please refer to the appendix for more cited studies. However, I think most of you have gotten the point. Eating fat or cholesterol does not increase blood cholesterol levels.

Myth 5: Cholesterol-lowering drugs are good for your health. They might lower cholesterol, but that doesn't necessarily do you any good. In fact, these drugs have yet to yield a reduction in heart attacks or stroke and may actually increase arteriosclerosis. You'll read all about this in chapter 8.

Five Cholesterol Facts

Fact 1: You will live longer with high cholesterol than low cholesterol. I know this statement is politically incorrect. However, scientific studies clearly show that people with high cholesterol live longer than those with low cholesterol. When you consider the important task that cholesterol plays in our bodies, it's not hard to imagine why. Consider the finding of Dr. Harlan Krumholz of the Department of Cardiovascular Medicine at Yale University. He reported in 1994 that old people with low cholesterol died twice as often from a heart attack as did old people with high cholesterol.[18]

The fact is that no one has ever died from high cholesterol. It has nothing to do with atherosclerosis or increased risk of death. But *low cholesterol* does increase the risk of premature death.

Fact 2: Low cholesterol can lead to depression and suicide. Remember Nathaniel Pritikin? Several studies show that among older adults, those with lowered cholesterol are more likely to suffer from depression. In fact, they are three times more likely to suffer from depression as are adults with normal cholesterol levels. And according to research published in *the British Medical Journal,* the lower the cholesterol, the more severe the depression.[19]

Low cholesterol levels have also been linked to an increased risk of committing suicide. Of the 300 victims of suicide evaluated by one study reported in *the British Medical Journal,* every one of them had low cholesterol levels.[20] Another study concluded that men whose cholesterol levels are lowered through the use of prescription medications double their chances of committing suicide.[21]

FACT 3: LOW CHOLESTEROL LEVELS ARE LINKED TO AN INCREASED RISK OF OTHER DEADLY ILLNESSES, INCLUDING CANCER. Men with total cholesterol levels below 160 double their risk of brain hemorrhage and increase their risk of liver, lung, and pancreatic cancer.[22]

FACT 4: WOMEN'S CHOLESTEROL LEVELS ARE ESSENTIALLY MEANINGLESS. So although we've seen that there is some sketchy and likely flawed "evidence" that high cholesterol levels could be linked to heart disease in men, *the Journal of the American Medical Association* reported in 1995 that there is *no* evidence linking high cholesterol levels in women with heart disease.[23] If you are female, the next time your doctor suggests you begin taking cholesterol-lowering drugs, please remind her of the medical studies that show total cholesterol levels as meaningless for women.

I'll repeat this again. Total cholesterol levels for women have been shown to be meaningless when related to heart disease! High levels have even been beneficial for some. Check out the title of this study published in 2003: "High Cholesterol May Protect Against Infections and Atherosclerosis."[24]

And Dr. Thomas Newman of the University of California at San Francisco has written extensively on cholesterol and heart disease, and he reports that cholesterol medications are less useful to women and may even increase their risk of death.[25] Women, please talk to your doctor about getting off your cholesterol-lowering medicine. It may save your life.

Fact 5: Cholesterol myths are the best thing to ever happen to drug companies. And recent guidelines have now lowered the acceptable limits for cholesterol in patients. Experts predict that the new guidelines will mean triple the prescriptions for statins and other lipid-lowering drugs. Pfizer (the makers of Lipitor) and other drug companies who push these drugs must be salivating.

In 2007, statin drugs were prescribed to over 13 million Americans, creating a $20 billion market in this country alone (Lipitor accounted for almost $10 billion), and there are an estimated 25 million users worldwide.[26]

So many doctors have bitten the hook of propaganda cast by the drug companies. They've been duped into believing that everyone needs to be on statin drugs. It's not as if these doctors are idiots. But the drug companies continue to churn out pseudoscientific studies (that must be later *investigated* in order to get at the truth) promoting the use of drug to lower cholesterol. In 2004, drug companies paid over $400 million to marketing firms who supplied ghostwriters to write and place articles in medical journals. Drug companies now pay for 62% of all articles that appear in medical journals, and 87% of FDA doctors receive money from drug companies—while the voiceless dying continue to take their pills as directed.

We have to face the facts, despite the cheerful commercials. Whatever the sentiments of their founders, drug companies survive by one tactic and one tactic only: selling as many of their drugs to as many people as possible. They aren't bashful about paying off doctors, ghostwriters, and even FDA officials to tow the line. They are happy to line their pockets while millions of Americans succumb to dangerous side effects, potentially worthless or harmful drugs, and skyrocketing medical costs.

For those of you still not convinced to talk to your doctor about abandoning your statin drug, read the next chapter. If you need more studies to sift through, please see the appendix.

Notes

1. T.B. Horwich et al., "Low Serum Total Cholesterol is Associated with Marked Increase in Mortality In Advanced Heart Failure," *Journal of Cardiac Failure* 8(4) (2002): 216–24.
2. T. Fujimoto, "Calcium Pump of the Plasma Membrane is Localized in Caveole," *Journal of Cellular Biology* 120 (1993): 1147–57.
3. Sherry Rogers, *The Cholesterol Hoax* (Syracuse: Prestige, 2008).
4. K.E. Landé and W.M. Sperry, "Human Atherosclerosis in Relation to the Cholesterol Content of the Blood Serum," *Archives of Pathology* 22 (1936): 301–12.
5. J.C. Paterson JC, R. Armstrong, and E.C. Armstrong, "Serum Lipid Levels and the Severity of Coronary and Cerebral Atherosclerosis in Adequately Nourished Men, 60 to 69 Years of Age," *Circulation* 27 (1963): 229–36.
6. F.M. Sacks et al., "Effect on Coronary Atherosclerosis of Decrease in Plasma Cholesterol Concentrations in Normocholesterolaemic Patients," *Lancet* 344 (1994): 1182–86.
7. "Profile of the Framingham Heart Study," web article (February 2006), www.framingham.com/heart/profile.htm.
8. *British Medical Journal,* "Rapid Responses to": Eric J G Sijbrands et al., "Mortality Over Two Centuries in Large Pedigree with Familial Hypercholesterolaemia: Family Tree Mortality Study," *British Medical Journal* 322 (2001): 1019–23, www.bmj.com/cgi/eletters/322/7293/1019.
9. H.M. Krumholz et al., "Lack of Association Between Cholesterol and Coronary Heart Disease Mortality and Morbidity and All-cause Mortality in Persons Older than 70 Years," *Journal of the American Medical Association* 272 (1994): 1335–40.
10. P.M. Riaker et al., "Comparison of C-Reactive Protein and Low Density Lipoprotein Cholesterol Levels in the Prediction of First Cardiovascular Events," *New England Journal of Medicine* 322(23) (June 7, 1990): 1635–41.
11. M. Sasahara et al., "Inhibition of Hypocholesterolemia-induced Atherosclerosis in Nonhuman Primate by Probucol 1: Is the Extent of Atherosclerosis Related to LDL Oxidation?" *Journal of Clinical Investigation* 94(1) (1994): 155–64.
12. P. Holvoet et al., "The Metabolic Syndrome, Circulating Oxidized LDL, and Risk of Myocardial Infarction in Well-Functioning Elderly People in the Health, Aging, and Body Composition Cohort," *Diabetes* 53(4) (April 1, 2004): 1068–73.
13. E. M. Kristenson et al., "Antioxidant State and Mortality from Coronary Heart Disease in Lithuanian and Swedish Men," *British Medical Journal* 314 (March, 1997): 629.
14. U. Ravnskov, "The Questionable Role of Saturated Fat and Polyunsaturated Fatty Acids in Cardiovascular Disease," *Journal of Clinical Epidemiology* 51,443–460,1998.

15. Jonny Bowden and Barry Sears, *Living the Low Carb Life: From Atkins to the Zone, Choosing the Diet That's Right for You* (Barnes & Noble Publishing, 2003), 204.
16. ibid.
17. A. B.Nichols et al., "Daily Nutritional Intake and Serum Lipid Levels: The Tecumseh study," *American Journal of Clinical Nutrition* 29 (1976): 1384–92.
18. H.M. Krumholz et al., "Lack of Association Between Cholesterol and Coronary Heart Disease Mortality and Morbidity and All-cause Mortality in Persons Older than 70 Years," *Journal of the American Medical Association* 272 (1994): 1335–40.
19. Bruno Bertozzi et al., correspondence, *British Medical Journal* 312 (1996): 1289–99.
20. M. Gallerani et al., "Serum Cholesterol Concentrations in Parasuicide," *British Medical Journal* 310 (1995): 1632–6.
21. G. Lindberg et al., "Low Serum Cholesterol Concentration and Short Term Mortality from Injuries in Men and Women," *British Medical Journal* 305 (1992): 277–9.
22. J.D. Neaton et al., "Serum Cholesterol Level and Mortality Findings for Men Screened in the Multiple Risk Factor Intervention Trial," *Archives of Internal Medicine* 152(7) (July 1992): 1490–1500.
23. Need Author Name, "Need Article Title," *Journal of the American Medical Association* 274(14) (1995): 1152–8.
24. U. Ravnskov, "High Cholesterol May Protect Against Infections and Atherosclerosis," *Quarterly Journal of Medicine* 96 (2003): 927–34.
25. Donald R. Davis, correspondence, *New England Journal of Medicine* 334(20) (1996): 1334.
26. Ingri Cassel, "The Horrors of Statin Drugs: The Misguided War on Cholesterol," *Idaho Observer* (October 2007), available at www.proliberty.com/observer/20071001.htm.

8

Medical Myths of Statin Drugs

THE MOST PRESCRIBED DRUGS IN THE WORLD, the cholesterol-lowering drugs known as statins have received scores of well-bought—oops, I mean, well-received—praise. Some medical folk have even suggested we start putting them in our drinking water. That would be nice, wouldn't it? Then we could all have amnesia, muscle pain, fatigue, and depression together! I'm sorry, but I just couldn't resist jumping to the punch line.

Unfortunately, it's no joke. Over the past 20 years, the pharmaceutical companies have promoted statin drugs with such fervor that they've now become household names: Lipitor, Zocor, Vytorin, Crestor, and others. They've enlisted scientists, advertising agencies, the media, and the medical profession in their cause to squash cholesterol levels. Sixteen million Americans now take Lipitor, the most popular statin, and drug-company officials claim that 36 million Americans are candidates for statin-drug therapy. Statin sales in the United States alone are over $26 billion a year. And the odd thing is that statins don't actually heal anything. All they do is shut down the liver enzyme reductase, which is needed for cholesterol production.

Four Statin Myths

Myth 1: Statin drugs save lives. Statin drugs have been hailed as the new wonder drugs for combating high cholesterol and heart disease because they appeared to be an improvement over older lipid-lowering drugs known as bile acid sequestrants (BASs). BASs have several unpleasant side effects, including nausea, indigestion, and constipation, and they are not very effective at lowering cholesterol levels. In contrast, statin drugs initially appeared to have no immediate side effects. And they are able to substantially lower cholesterol levels by up to 50 points. And what's more, for patients who have already had a heart attack, statins lower the their risk of dying from another one by a full 1.1%! *Wait a minute, that's not as impressive as they make it sound on TV.*

In the CARE trial, the odds of escaping death from a heart attack in five years for a patient with manifest heart disease were 94.3%. Not bad. This improved to 95.4% with statin treatment. This is a difference of 1.1 percent.[1]

You mean to tell me that all this fuss about statin medications has been over the fact that those who had already had a heart attack and were now taking statins were 1.1% less likely to die from another heart attack than those not who had already had a heart attack and were not taking statins?

Yep. I'm afraid so. In the scientific papers and in the drug advertisements, these small effects are translated into big claims. In the WOSCOPS trial, for instance, it is said that mortality was lowered with statin drugs by 25%, because the difference between a mortality of 1.6% in the control group and 1.2% in the treatment group is 25%.[2] Still, the difference between the two groups is less than 1/2 of 1%! But "25%" sounds a lot better.

How does this misinformation happen? The public and the medical profession have been bamboozled by the legions of drug reps, billion-dollar ad campaigns, and "creative" statistics. Every weekday, some 38,000 Pfizer sales reps, a group roughly the size of three army divisions, make their pitches around the globe. They're armed with briefcases full of free drug samples, reams of manipulated clinical data, and lavish expense accounts for wining and dining doctors and their staffs. Pfizer is now running full-page Lipitor ads in numerous papers, including *the New York Times* and *USA Today.* The ads feature Dr. Robert Jarvik, inventor of the artificial heart, and read, "In patients with multiple risk factors for heart disease, Lipitor reduces risk of heart attack by 36%*." The noteworthy part of this ad is the asterisk. It leads to a little note that discloses, "That means in a large clinical study, 3% of patients taking a sugar pill or placebo had a heart attack compared to 2% of patients taking Lipitor." Not quite as impressive when you put it that way.

Another Jarvik Lipitor ad in the Times proclaims, "In patients with type-2 diabetes, Lipitor reduces risk of stroke by 48%* if you also have at least one other risk factor for heart disease." The asterisk explanation here reads, "That means in a large clinical study, 2.8% of patients taking a sugar pill or placebo had a stroke compared to 1.5% of patients taking Lipitor."

We're spending $26 billion a year for a 1%–2% decreased risk for heart attack or stroke? That's what all the fuss is about? It almost seems like snake oil. Yet some doctors are recommending we put statins in the drinking water. Others are even suggesting that infants with a family history of heart disease take statins as a preventative measure.

And perhaps your doctor, convinced that statin drugs are harmless, routinely prescribes them for anyone with a cholesterol level above 200. He might even cite a number of studies in which statin use has lowered the number of heart attack deaths compared to controls. But if we look a little deeper into these studies, we see that statin medications do not *significantly* reduce the risk, and some studies have shown no improvement at all. A meta-analysis of 26 controlled cholesterol-lowering trials found an *equal* number of cardiovascular deaths in the treatment and control groups.[3] And by reducing your cholesterol, statins can actually *increase* your risk of death overall.

A 2001 study called the Honolulu Heart Program was primarily concerned with cholesterol and the elderly. To quote from the report—which appeared in *the Lancet*— "Our data accords with previous findings of increased mortality in elderly people with low serum cholesterol, and show that long-term persistence of low cholesterol concentration actually increases risk of death."

Researchers went on to say, "Although our results lend support to previous findings that low serum cholesterol imparts a poor outlook when compared with higher concentrations of cholesterol in elderly people, our data also suggest that those individuals with a low serum cholesterol maintained over a 20-year period will have the worst outlook for all-cause mortality."[4] Read that again. That *has* to hurt the "let's put statins in the drinking water" argument.[5]

A 2004 study found that the statin drug Zocor does not decrease heart attacks, stroke, or death at all. Worse, one in 250 patients in the study who took the highest dose of Zocor had serious muscle-weakening side effects,[6] which in rare cases can be lethal (more about this in "Myth 5," below).

So the question isn't, "Do statin drugs reduce the incidence of certain kinds of deaths for certain kinds of people?" The real question is this: "Do statin drugs reduce deaths?" That would be *my* definition of life-saving. Whether it's from heart attack or side effects, death is death, friend. And we want to avoid it.

Myth 2: The makers of statin drugs have your health as their first priority. Doubt it. Consider the two-year ENHANCE trial: The long-awaited results of this recent trial of the cholesterol-lowering drug Vytorin (ever heard of it? Those fun little commercials where the relatives look like the food?) revealed that it *isn't* any more effective than the older (and a lot cheaper) statin drugs. In fact, those taking Vytorin had a little bit *more* plaque buildup during the trial than those on the statin drug alone.[7] Oddly enough, the makers of this drug, Merck and Schering-Plough, suppressed the findings for 20 months and continued to aggressively market the product during that time. They might never have revealed the results if not for pressure to do so from an article in the *New York Times* as well as a Congressional inquiry.

The makers of Vytorin now claim that they had nothing to hide. It's tough to believe that they weren't just a little reluctant to publish their highly anticipated study. The news that their new drug, which retails for $100 a month (and did $2 billion in sales in 2007) was clinically inferior to a generic statin costing less than $20 a month obviously wasn't what their stockholders wanted to hear. And I can understand their concern. They had invested a lot of money in the success of this drug. Merck and Schering-Plough had teamed up to fight the statin Goliath, Pfizer, and bring down its Lipitor Empire! I for one do not want my heart health getting caught up in their drug war.

Now, Merck and Schering-Plough are running full-page ads daily in *the Times* and *the Wall Street Journal,* warning people not to be mislead by a single study and to continue taking Vytorin. The advice was backed by the American Heart Association, which—by the way—*the Times* reported receives nearly $2 million a year from Merck and Schering-Plough Pharmaceuticals.[8]

Dr. Steven Nissen, director of cardiovascular medicine at the Cleveland Clinic, responded angrily to the news of Vytorin's failure. "We are supposed to continue giving these drugs on faith for the next four or five years in the hope that they work," he said. "That makes no sense. We practice evidence-based medicine, and right now the only evidence we have suggests that [Vytorin adds] nothing [to traditional statins] in terms of health benefits."[9] I practice evidence-based medicine, too, and I couldn't agree more.

Other statins have completely bitten the dust in the past couple of years. Pfizer's trial of its drug torcetrapib, which raises HDL and lowers LDL, had to be stopped in 2006 because the drug caused heart attacks and strokes.[10]

All the efforts of the drug companies are paying off. From the Washington Post comes this report on a drug study: " 'The findings should prompt doctors to give much higher doses of drugs known as statins to hundreds of thousands of patients who already have severe heart problems,' experts said. 'In addition, it will probably encourage physicians to start giving the medications to millions of healthy people who are not yet on them and to boost dosages for some of those already taking them to lower their cholesterol even more.' "[11]

The last line of this quote should send shivers through every taxpayer in America. Why? Because it will be the taxpayers who pay for all those Medicaid and Medicare prescriptions. Worse, we'll be paying for all the costs associated with the drug-induced side effects of the statin medications.

"Statins make victims—a lot of victims—and by now it's pretty clear how they do it," is the bold comment of cardiologist Dr. Peter Langsjoen from Tyler, Texas. "We are at the beginning of the biggest medical tragedy that mankind ever witnessed," Langsjoen says. "Never before in history has the medical establishment knowingly created a life-threatening nutrient deficiency in millions of otherwise healthy people, only to sit back with arrogance and horrific irresponsibility and watch to see what happens. I cannot help to view my once great profession with a mixture of sorrow and contempt."[12]

The AMA's Code of Medical Ethics requires that patients receive informed consent about all reasonably effective treatments: "The patient's right of self-decision can be effectively exercised only if the patient possesses enough information to enable an intelligent choice. The physician has an ethical obligation to help the patient make choices from among the therapeutic alternatives consistent with good medical practice."[13] Has your doctor informed you about the potential side effects of your statin medications?

Myth 3: Statins reduce plaque in your arteries. A study published in the *American Journal of Cardiology* casts serious doubts on the commonly held belief that lowering your LDL-cholesterol, the so-called bad cholesterol, is the most effective way to reduced arterial plaque. On average, subjects in both groups (those taking high and low doses of satin medications) showed a 9.2% increase in plaque buildup.[14]

In other words, it didn't matter how much or how little statin medication they took, or how much their cholesterol levels were lowered. They still had an increase in plaque! This should put the nail in the coffin of the cholesterol theory. Lowering cholesterol doesn't prevent plaque formation, because cholesterol isn't the cause of arteriosclerosis (see chapter 7).

Myth 4: Statins don't have serious side effects. If you've read chapter 7, you probably have a knowing suspicion that this is one dangerous myth. Let's look at each of these "minor" side effects in detail.

Coenzyme Q10 Deficiency and Muscle Death

First, statins deplete your body of coenzyme Q10 (CoQ10). This is an enzyme that works with other enzymes to keep the body's metabolic functions working at optimal levels. Small amounts of CoQ10 are found in foods (such as meat and seafood). However, blood levels of CoQ10 decrease with age, hypertension, statin use, diabetes, and atherosclerosis.

CoQ10's main purpose is to increase the function of the mitochondria, the power plants of each cell. A CoQ10 deficiency can lead to angina, hypertension, and accelerated aging. But most notably, CoQ10 is vital to the formation of healthy elastin and collagen, so another potentially fatal effect of a CoQ10 deficiency is muscle wasting, which can lead to weakness, severe fatigue and back pain, heart failure (the heart is a muscle, after all), neuropathy, inflammation of the tendons and ligaments (often leading to rupture), and fibromyalgia-like symptoms. The statin drug Baycol was withdrawn because it was linked to 100 deaths from rhabdomyolysis (muscle death) and over 1,100 cases of muscle weakness. Drug company Bayer, maker of Baycol, has 8,400 resulting law suits against it.

But Baycol is not the only statin to cause rhabdomyolysis. The other statins still pose a rare risk for this disorder, especially at daily doses of 80 mg. or more. Information in the following chart is drawn from *MedWatch* spontaneous "Adverse Event Reports" for one month in the United States.[15]

Number of Rhabdomyolysis Events Reported

- Zocor : 278
- Lipitor: 100
- Pravachol: 62
- Lescol: 11
- Baycol: 1,100
- Mevacor: 97
- Lopid: 35

The most common indication of this terrible illness of rhabdomyolysis is muscle pain and weakness, most likely due to the depletion of CoQ10, as explained above. The drug-insert literature for statin drugs downplays the muscle pain and weakness and suggests that they occur in about 2% of the patients taking statin drugs. However, one study found that 98% of patients taking Lipitor and 1/3 of the patients taking Mevachor (a lower-dose statin) suffered from muscle problems.[16] It's become so common that any time one of my patients complains of muscle pain, I always ask if they are taking a statin drug. And sadly, many of the patients who consult me for muscle pain—including those with fibromyalgia—have never been told that their statin drugs may be causing their problem.

I had one patient who, almost immediately after starting Zocor, started experiencing diffuse muscle pain. He had regular x-rays, an MRI, a bone scan, several blood workups, and finally a nerve-conduction study. All were normal. One doctor he consulted before seeing me said his liver enzymes were normal and it must be the diuretic he was taking. He was prescribed NSAID medication for his chronic pain, but it caused him to start having reflux, so he was placed on Nexium. Then he began having a good deal of fatigue. The Nexium was doing such a good job of blocking his stomach acid that he couldn't absorb vitamin B12, and that was knocking out his energy, along with the statin-induced CoQ10 deficiency. I was able to help this patient make a pretty speedy recovery. It took a little time to wean off these medications, but once he did, his battle with muscle pain, fatigue, and reflux disappeared overnight.

The blood test for rhabdomyolysis is elevated levels of a chemical called creatine kinase (CK). But some statin-drug patients experience pain and fatigue even though they have normal CK levels.[17] If you are experiencing muscle pain or weakness on your statin drug, keep after your doctor until she addresses your symptoms! But you don't have to consult your doctor before starting to supplement with CoQ10, which your body is likely craving. Individuals taking statin medications should replace their CoQ10 by taking a minimum of 100 mg. a day. To combat muscle aches and pains, as much as 200 mg. a day may be needed.

Other symptoms of a CoQ10 deficiency include gum disease, memory loss, depression, and even some forms of cancer.

Polyneuropathy

Another potentially life-altering effect of statin drugs concerns your neurological system. Polyneuropathy, also known as peripheral neuropathy, is characterized by neurological inflammation that causes weakness, tingling, and pain in the hands and feet. Chronic inflammatory polyneuropathy is a disorder involving slowly progressive or repeated episodes of loss of movement or sensation, caused by inflammation of multiple nerves. Use of statin drugs causes a 14-fold increase in the risk of developing polyneuropathy.[18]

Symptoms of polyneuropathy include weakness, pain, burning, tingling, numbness, or paralysis in the arms and hands, legs and feet, or the face; difficulty walking or moving; difficulty swallowing or speaking; voice hoarseness or changes; muscle contractions and atrophy; joint pain; fatigue; bowel or bladder dysfunction; and difficulty breathing.

I often see patients with statin-induced polyneuropathy. Many of them have undergone a battery of neurological tests. When the tests come back normal, they are placed on Neurontin, which is now being used to block nerve-related pain. But Neurontin has several side effects, including dizziness, weakness, fatigue, double-vision, abnormal eyeball movement, tremors, weight gain, back pain, constipation, muscle aches, memory loss, depression, abnormal thinking, itching, twitching, and runny nose. As you can see, Neurontin isn't a drug you want to be taking, especially to cover up the side effects of your statin medication.

A Denmark study that evaluated 500,000 patients found that people who took statins were more likely to develop polyneuropathy. Taking statins for one year raised the risk of nerve damage by about 15%—about one case for every 2,200 patients. For those who took statins for two or more years, the risk rose to 26%.[19,20] This might not seem like a big risk. But we're talking about nerve damage! All for a drug that isn't proven to help your heart anyway.

Congestive Heart Failure

Lastly, I don't want to start any conspiracy theories, but this is an interesting observation: The incidence of congestive heart failure (CHF) has steadily increased since the introduction of statin drugs. In fact, while heart attacks have slightly declined, CHF has more than doubled since 1989, and statins were first prescribed in 1987.[21]

Cardiologist Peter Langsjoen studied 20 patients with completely normal heart function. Within six months of starting on 20 mg. of Lipitor a day, 2/3 of the patients had heart abnormalities. According to Langsjoen, this malfunction was due to CoQ10 depletion.[22]

Without CoQ10, the cell's mitochondria are inhibited from producing energy, and this leads to muscle pain and weakness. The heart muscle is especially susceptible to this deprivation, because it uses so much energy.[23] In spite of the fact that biochemistry, something all doctors learned (through some evidently forgot), shows the importance of CoQ10 for proper heart-muscle function, those with CHF are routinely placed on statin medications. This is pure insanity.

Lipitor may be contributing to cardiovascular disease in another way, as it decreases vitamin E and the vitamin A precursor, beta carotene, by 28%.[24] We've already seen how important vitamin E is in regard to heart health.

Statin drugs also deplete folic acid, a B vitamin that protects our genes from oxidation (damage) from environmental toxins. Folic acid, as we'll see later, plays a critical role in reducing homocysteine (a marker for increased risk of heart disease and stroke).

Memory Loss

What about my comment in the first paragraph about amnesia? Former astronaut Dr. Duane Graveline describes his complete memory loss—due to the side effects of Lipitor—in his book, *Lipitor: Thief of Memory.* Unfortunately, Dr. Graveline is only one in a growing number of individuals who have experienced memory loss caused by statin medications. Often these people are told by their doctors that they are just getting older. Since when is extensive memory loss a normal part of the aging process? I wonder how many older adults diagnosed with presenile dementia are really suffering from "statin disease"? Statin drugs have even been linked to Alzheimer's disease.[25]

Dizziness

Dizziness is also commonly associated with statin use. Combine this with an elderly patient, and you have a hip fracture in the making.

Cancer

I've already reported on the potential risk of statin use and cancer. An article published in the *Journal of the American Medical Association* reveals that in *every* study to date with rodents, statins have caused cancer.[26] In the previously mentioned CARE trial, breast cancer rates of those taking a statin went up 1500%.[27]

Depression and Suicide

I've also already discussed how low cholesterol levels are associated with depression and suicide. Consequently, depression is a common side effect in those taking statin medications. One study showed that one out of three statin users suffered from low moods.[28] Being told that your heart is at risk is depressing enough. Blasting cholesterol with high doses of statin drugs only increases the risk of depression. Before you refill your Paxil prescription, I suggest you have your cholesterol checked, and by all means, reconsider taking statin medications.

For those of you who need further proof that statin drugs are dangerous, increase mortality rates, and may be worthless, please refer to additional studies listed in the appendix.

The List Goes On

Statin drugs deplete the mineral selenium, a vital nutrient for proper immune function. Low selenium levels can cause hypothyroid symptoms: fatigue, weight gain, depression, high blood pressure, hair loss, and poor immune function.

When there isn't enough cholesterol (due to cholesterol-lowering statins), the electrically charged channels that regulate cellular calcium become clogged. These calcium pumps control how much calcium gets into and out of the cell. When calcium becomes stuck inside the cells, it can trigger several unwanted symptoms—irregular heartbeat, high blood pressure, chest pain, and…you guessed it…congestive heart failure.[29]

We'll look closer at calcium-channel-blocking drugs later in the book.

Notes

1. F.M. Sacks et al., "The Effect of Pravastatin on Coronary Events After Myocardial Infarction in Patients with Average Cholesterol Levels," *New England Journal of Medicine* 335 (1996): 1001–9.
2. Uffe Ravnskov, *The Cholesterol Myths* (Washington: New Trends, 2000).
3. U. Ravnskov, "Cholesterol Lowering Trials in Coronary Heart Disease: Frequency of Citation and Outcome," *British Medical Journal* 305 (1992): 15–19.
4. I.J. Schatz et al., "Cholesterol and All Cause Mortality in Elderly People in the Honolulu Heart Program: A Cohort Study," *Lancet* 358 (2001): 351–355.
5. G.G. Schwartz and et al., "Effects of Atorvastatin on Early Recurrent Ischemic Events," *Journal of the American Medical Association* 285 (2001): 1711–8.
6. J.A. de Lemos, "Early Intensive vs. a Delayed Conservative Simvastatin Strategy in Patients with Acute Coronary Syndromes: Phase Z of the A to Z Trial," *Journal of the American Medical Association* 292 (2004): 1307–1316.
7. J. Kastelein et al., "Simvastatin With or Without Ezetimibe in Familial Hypercholesterolemia," *New England Journal of Medicine* 358 (2008): 1431–43.
8. Melissa Healy, "Vytorin Study Raises Questions About Cholesterol's Import," *HealthFacts* (February, 2008).
9. Salynn Boyles, "Study Casts Doubts on Vytorin, Zetia: Cholesterol-Lowering Drugs May Not Reduce Plaque Buildup," *WebMD Health News* (January 15, 2008), www.webmd.com/cholesterol-management/news/20080115/study-casts-doubts-on-vytorin-zetia.
10. Alex Berenson, "Pfizer Drug Dealt Death Blow in Testing," *New York Times* (November 1, 2006).
11. Elizabeth Scherdt, "The Struggles of Older Drivers," letter, *Washington Post* (June 21, 2003).
12. Melchior Meijer, "Statins—Miracle Drug or Tragedy?," The International Network of Cholesterol Skeptics, web article, www.thincs.org/melchior1.htm.
13. *Code of Medical Ethics* available at www.ama-assn.org/ama/pub/category/2498.html.
14. H.S. Hecht et al., "Relation of Aggressiveness of Lipid-lowering Treatment to Changes in Calcified Plaque Burden by Electron Beam Tomography," *American Journal of Cardiology* 92 (2003): 334–6.
15. The Fibonacci Group, *MedWatch (*from data collected August 2001).
16. Eleanor Laise, "The Lipitor Dilemma," *Smart Money: The Wall Street Journal Magazine of Personal Business* (November 2003).
17. Beatrice A. Golomb, "Questions about STATINS," Cardio Files, entry on Q-and-A web forum (March 7, 2002), www.cardiofiles.net/forums/heart-attacks-and-diseases/8253-questions-about-statins.html. See more

from Golomb through the University of California at San Diego's Statin Effects Study, www.statineffects.com/info.

18. D. Gaist et al., "Statins and Risk of Polyneuropathy: A Case Study," *Neurology* 58(9) (2002): 1333–7.
19. ibid.
20. ibid.
21. P.H. Langsjoen, "The clinical Use of HMG CoA-reductase Inhibitors (Statins) and the Associated Depletion of the Essential Co-factor coenzyme Q10: a Review of Pertinent Human and Animal Data," available www.fda.gov/ohrms/dockets/dailys/02/May02/052902/02p-0244-cp00001-02-Exhibit_A-vol1.pdf.
22. Melchior Meijer, "Statins—Miracle Drug or Tragedy?," The International Network of Cholesterol Skeptics, web article, www.thincs.org/melchior1.htm.
23. Eleanor Laise, "The Lipitor Dilemma," Smart Money (November 2003).
24. Sherry Rogers, *The Cholesterol Hoax* (Syracuse: Prestige, 2008), 7.
25. ibid., 12.
26. T.B. Newman and S.B. Hulley, "Carcinogenicity of Lipid-lowering Drugs" *Journal of the American Medical Association* 27 (1996): 55–60.
27. F.M. Sacks et al., "The Effects of Pravastatin on Coronary Events After Myocardial Infarction in Patients with Average Cholesterol Levels," *New England Journal of Medicine* 385 (1996): 1001–9.
28. K. Morales et al., "Simvastatin Causes Changes in Affective Processes in Elderly Volunteers," *Journal of the American Geriatric Society* 54 (January 2006): 7–76.
29. T. Fujimoto, "Calcium Pump of Plasma Membrane is Localized in Caveolae," *Journal of Cellular Biology* 120 (1993): 1147–57.

9

Safe and Effective Alternative Treatments

Many conventional medical doctors are quick to point out that over-the-counter supplements are not regulated by the Food and Drug Administration (FDA). This is the same FDA that regulates the prescription drug industry, which we now know is associated with over 100,000 deaths each year. This is the same FDA that fought tooth-and-nail to prevent the public from finding out about the increased risk of suicide in children on antidepressant medications. This is the same organization that tried to squelch one of their own, Dr. David Graham, from blowing the whistle on Vioxx. If Dr. Graham had not presented his findings that Vioxx had already been linked to over 27,000 heart attack deaths (according to the *FDA),* that dangerous medication would still be on the market.

And this is the same FDA that has recently declined a petition by well-known author Dr. Julien Whitaker (and others) to place warning labels on statin medications advising of stain-induced CoQ10 deficiencies. This organization—paid for by tax dollars and entrusted to protect the citizens of the United States—has turned the other way in the face of insurmountable evidence that statin medications cause CoQ10 deficiencies.

Many conventional doctors simply say, "There are no studies to prove that supplements work." That one is easy to disprove. There are *numerous* studies that positively show that a wide assortment of nutritional supplements are as or more effective—and certainly safer—than prescription medications. Dr. Mark Houston, associate clinical professor of medicine at Vanderbilt University School of Medicine, points out that there are well over 1,000 studies that validate the use of natural medicines to reverse hypertension alone.[1] But even if doctors aren't aware of these studies, they simply *can't* claim ignorance of what Dr. Angell, past editor of the *New England Journal of Medicine,* has begun to point out: much of what is published in scientific journals has been funded, and meticulously overseen, by drug companies. Surely these studies aren't any *more* trustworthy than the tests done on inexpensive and easy-to-produce natural remedies. Let's look at some of these remedies that have been tested and found to be beneficial for treating heart disease and hypertension.

Fish Oil

The American Heart Association reported findings that fish-oil supplements drastically reduce the risk of sudden death from heart attack and/or stroke. The study consisted of 11,323 patients who had suffered a heart attack within the previous three months. One group was supplemented with 1,000 mg. of fish oil a day. After only three months, there was an incredible 41% reduction in the risk of sudden death. At the end of the three-and-a-half-year study, those receiving fish-oil supplementation were 45% less likely to die from a heart-related disease.[2]

For nearly two decades, the FDA prevented this lifesaving information from reaching the public, even though the research clearly shows the benefits of consuming omega-3 (fish) oils. The FDA fought for seven years, spending millions of taxpayer dollars, to prevent this statement from appearing on nutritional-supplement labels: "Consumption of omega-3 fatty acids may reduce the risk of coronary heart disease." After losing a lawsuit brought against them, the FDA finally had no choice but to allow the use of this statement.

It wasn't that long ago that the U.S. government, along with the AMA and the FDA, made it illegal to even imply that essential fatty acids (such as omega-3 oils) had any relationship to diseases of the heart and arteries. To do so was a criminal offense! Finally, in May of 2003, The White House urged health agencies to encourage Americans to increase their consumption of foods rich in omega-3 fatty acids and to decrease their intake of harmful trans fatty acids.[3]

It is now estimated that if every American regularly took fish-oil supplements or consumed two servings of cold-water fish a week, it would save 150,000 lives a year.

Magnesium

Magnesium is an essential mineral involved in over 300 bodily enzymatic processes. It is responsible for proper enzyme activity and transmission of muscle and nerve impulses, and it aids in maintaining a proper pH balance. It helps metabolize carbohydrates, proteins, and fats into energy. It helps synthesize the genetic material in cells and remove toxic substances, such as aluminum and ammonia, from the body. Adequate amounts of magnesium are *needed* for proper heart function, and a deficiency of magnesium may increase your risk of heart disease from free-radical damage.

How it helps your heart: Magnesium can actually serve as treatment of your current heart condition. If you heart overworked? Magnesium is a natural sedative that relaxes muscles. The heart (which is mostly muscle) and the smooth muscle contained in blood-vessel lining are dependent on magnesium. A deficiency leads to muscle spasms or contractions. Supplementing with magnesium can correct this deficiency.

Also, recall that beta-blocker medications block the effects of adrenaline (and norepinephrine) on a cell's beta-receptors. This slows the nerve impulses that stimulate the heart, so the heart does not work as hard. Magnesium acts like a natural beta blocker by inhibiting these stimulatory hormones. Fortunately, magnesium does not cause fatigue or the other symptoms associated with prescription beta blockers.[4]

Magnesium also acts as a natural calcium-channel blocker. The more calcium found within a muscle cell, the more tense or tight that muscle becomes. So calcium-channel blockers try to prevent too much calcium from entering the cell membrane through the cell's calcium channels. But what many doctors overlook is that these calcium channels are *guarded* by a magnesium valve. If a person is deficient in magnesium, calcium ions are able to infiltrate cells and cause muscle (such as heart) contraction. The more magnesium found within a muscle cell, the more relaxed the muscle becomes. And a relaxed heart is a happy heart.

Some studies show that those with mitral valve prolapse (MVP) are deficient in magnesium.[5] Others show that magnesium reduces the symptoms of MVP, including palpitations, chest pain, and fatigue.[6] Magnesium deficiency is also linked to stoke, since too little of it can lead to spasms in the arteries (remember, blood vessels are dependent on adequate levels of magnesium in order to relax). Dozens of research papers have been written on how a magnesium deficiency can trigger these arterial spasms, which can lead to stroke.[7] These spasms may be felt as chest pain, leg cramps, eye twitching, or TIAs (transient ischemic attacks).

More About Magnesium Deficiency

"Since the turn of this century, there has been a steady and progressive decline of dietary magnesium intake to where much of the Western World population is ingesting less than an optimum RDA."[8] Researchers at the Department of Physiology, State University of New York's Health Science Center at Brooklyn have shown that the U.S. population doesn't get the recommended daily allowance of magnesium. The RDA for magnesium is 400 mg. a day. The estimated intake in the United States is 300 mg. a day. But studies show as much as three times this amount may be needed by the general population, especially by those predisposed to cardiac disease states.[9]

Magnesium has been consistently depleted in our soils. It has been further depleted in plants by the use of potassium-and phosphorus-containing fertilizers, which reduce the plant's ability to uptake magnesium. Food processing removes magnesium even further, while our high-carbohydrate and high-fat diets *increase* the need for magnesium. If you take diuretic medications or inject insulin, these can further deplete your total body magnesium.

Recent research in France and several other European countries gives a clue concerning the role magnesium plays in the transmission of hormones (such as insulin, thyroid, estrogen, testosterone, DHEA, etc.), neurotransmitters (such as dopamine, catecholamines, serotonin, GABA, etc.), minerals, and mineral electrolytes.

This research concludes that it is the magnesium status of the body that controls cell-membrane potential. If there is not enough magnesium, these substances can't even do their jobs. For instance, if magnesium is insufficient, potassium and calcium will be lost in the urine, and further calcium will be deposited in the soft tissues (kidneys, arteries, joints, brain, etc.),[10] leading to arteriosclerosis, or calcified arteries.

A deficiency in magnesium can also cause depression, muscle cramps, high blood pressure, heart disease and arrhythmia, constipation, insomnia, loss of hair, confusion, personality disorders, swollen gums, and loss of appetite. And new studies are validating what many nutrition-oriented physicians have known for years: a magnesium deficiency can trigger migraine headaches.[11]

Other uses of magnesium include treating muscle spasms, anxiety, depression, insomnia, and constipation. It also helps with intermittent claudication (a condition caused by a restriction of blood flow) and helps relax constricted bronchial tubes associated with asthma. High intake of calcium may reduce magnesium absorption. Simple sugars and stress deplete the body of magnesium.[12]

Dosage: Ideally, you should be taking a good comprehensive multivitamin and mineral supplement daily that contains 400–600 mg. of magnesium. I prefer my patients take magnesium chelate, citrate, or taurate, as these seem be absorbed the best. I find that individuals who use less-expensive magnesium oxide increase the risk of abdominal discomfort and loose bowel movements.

Toxicity: Magnesium supplemented above 600 mg. can cause loose stools and diarrhea, but this is quickly remedied by decreasing the dosage.

COENZME Q10

Discovered by researchers at the University of Wisconsin in 1957, coenzyme Q10 (CoQ10) is an essential nutrient for proper cardiovascular function and a powerful antioxidant. It's even been shown effective in some cases in returning decreased heart function to normal! This is especially true when discussing congestive heart failure.[13]

CoQ10 is also known as ubiquinone, from the word *ubiquitous,* meaning "found everywhere." That's because CoQ10 is found in every cell in the body. But it's more abundant in some cells and organs than others. Its primary function is to provide cellular energy, so CoQ10 tends to congregate in the organs that need the most energy, such as the heart and liver. In each cell, there are organelles (small organ cells) known as mitochondria. Mitochondria are similar to a car's cylinders; they allow a chain of chemical reactions to create a spark. This spark generates 95% of the body's energy. So without CoQ10, there is practically no cellular energy!

The body can't manufacture CoQ10; we must obtain it from the foods we eat. Meat, dairy, and certain vegetables like spinach and broccoli contain the highest concentrations of CoQ10. However, obtaining adequate CoQ10 through diet is a challenge for most adults. It takes a pound of sardines, or 2.5 pounds of peanuts to provide about 30 mg. of CoQ10. This is the very minimum of the recommended daily allowance. In reality, the typical daily intake of CoQ10 from dietary sources is 3–5 mg. This paltry amount isn't anywhere near the level required to significantly raise blood and tissue levels of the enzyme. As we age, we tend to absorb and utilize less CoQ10, though our need for it increases. This is most likely due to an increase in the amount of free radicals that our aging bodies generate.

How it helps your heart: The importance of CoQ10 to maintain optimal health can't be overstated. A growing body of research shows that it may benefit those with a number of health issues such as diabetes, periodontal disease, chronic fatigue, migraine headaches, skin cancers, infertility, immune dysfunction, asthma, muscular dystrophy, Alzheimer's disease, Parkinson's disease, and of course, cardiovascular disease.

The cardiovascular system is especially vulnerable to CoQ10 deficiencies, since the heart consumes huge amounts of CoQ10-initiated energy (remember that the muscles of the heart contract and relax some 100,000 times a day, pumping blood through 60,000 miles of arteries and veins with each beat).

Researchers investigating CoQ10 have estimated that as little as a 25% reduction in bodily CoQ10 will trigger various disease processes, including high blood pressure, coronary artery disease, cancer, and immune system dysfunction.[14] So an already low CoQ10 level combined with statin medication is a recipe for disaster. (For more about how stain drugs decrease CoQ10, see chapter 8.) What's more, the biosynthesis of CoQ10 from the amino acid tyrosine is a complex, highly vulnerable, 17-step process. It requires at least seven vitamins (B2, B3, B6, folic acid, B12, C, and B5) and several trace elements. Most American diets are deficient in at least one—if not many—of these cofactors for making CoQ10 (71% are deficient in B6 alone).

Dr. Karl Folkers and fellow researchers at the University of Texas are credited with identifying the importance of CoQ10 in bodily functions. Folkers has been honored with the Priestly Medal—the highest award bestowed by the American Chemical Society—for his work with CoQ10, vitamin B6, and vitamin B12. In his acceptance for the Priestly Medal, Folkers pointed out that CoQ10 therapy was a major advancement in the treatment of heart disease. He believes that suboptimal nutrient intake is almost universal in people, and these deficiencies prevent the biosynthesis of CoQ10. He suggests that since the average, "normal" levels of CoQ10 are really suboptimal, the very low levels observed in advanced disease states represent only the tip of the deficiency. Given the added stress posed in today's society and the need for an ever-increasing amount of antioxidants to counter this tress, could it be that many of our chronic illnesses are due to suboptimal levels of CoQ10?

For instance, in one of the studies cited by Dr. Folkers, those treated over a three-year period with CoQ10 and conventional medical therapies had a 75% survival rate compared to a 25% survival rate for those who used conventional drug therapy alone. Dr. Folkers went on to say, "I believe it is quite possible that cardiovascular disease may be significantly caused by a deficiency of CoQ10. CoQ10 is known to be deficient in congestive heart failure, with the degree of deficiency in blood and cardiac tissue correlating with the severity of the CHF."[15]

A group of class-IV (terminal) congestive-heart-failure patients were supplemented with CoQ10 in addition to their prescription medications. Sadly, class-IV patients normally live only a matter of days. But 71% of those taking the CoQ10 survived one year, and 62% survived two years![16]

Administering CoQ10 (50–150 mg. daily) for 90 days to 2,664 patients in congestive heart failure resulted in the following improvement in symptoms: 78% improvement in cyanosis (bluish skin color); 79% in edema, 78% in pulmonary crackle, 53% in dyspnea (poor breathing), 75% in palpitations, 80% in sweating, 63% in arrhythmia (irregular heartbeats), and 73% in vertigo.[17]

Research shows that taking 100–225 mg. of CoQ10 a day can reduce high systolic blood pressure by an average of 15 points and high diastolic pressure an average of 10 points. And more than half of patients receiving 225 mg. per day were able to terminate the use of 1–3 of their antihypertensive medications.[18]

Mitral valve prolapse is a common condition associated with a heart murmur. It is often asymptomatic but can produce chest pain, arrhythmia, or leakage of the valve, leading to congestive heart disease. One study showed that when children with mitral valve prolapse received CoQ10 (2 mg./kg. per day) for eight weeks, heart function returned to normal in seven of the eight children; *not one* of the placebo-treated patients improved. Relapse of symptoms was common among those who stopped taking the supplement within 12–17 months but rarely occurred in those who took CoQ10 for 19 months or more.[19]

In spite of all these accolades, there is a good chance that you—an American reader concerned about your heart—have never heard of this enzyme.

Dosage: I recommend my patients take a minimum of 50 mg. of high-quality CoQ10 a day for prevention or 100–200 mg. a day for treatment of coronary heart disease and associated high blood pressure. Patients in treatment for heart disease will need to take at least 100 mg. a day indefinitely, as symptoms of heart disease will usually return within two years of discontinuing therapy.

Until recently, CoQ10 was a prescription medication in Japan. It is quite popular there, with hundreds of commercial CoQ10 preparations from more than 80 different pharmaceutical companies. Over 12 million Japanese (approximately 10% of the population) take CoQ10 on a regular basis to prevent and treat heart disease. This number is rapidly growing, since recent laws now allow CoQ10 to be sold over-the-counter. Since Japanese physicians have a long track record of using CoQ10, 75% of all supplemental CoQ10 comes from Japan. The high-quality Japanese CoQ10 is fairly expensive, but venders and manufacturers predict that the price will eventually come down as Japanese manufacturers increase their capacity to meet the growing demand.

As for the American market, CoQ10 can cost as little as pennies per tablet. However, these cheaper forms are cheap for a reason. They use inferior CoQ10, usually loaded with fillers and additives. Pure, high-quality CoQ10 comes from Japan. It costs more but yields better results. Choose melting tabs, gel caps, or chewables of CoQ10; tablets require binders that restrict the enzyme's absorption. You can order good CoQ10 from Douglas Laboratories or my office (see the appendix for ordering information).

Vitamin E

Vitamin E is a fat-soluble vitamin and a powerful antioxidant that has been touted for its numerous potential health benefits. It can help you stay healthy and fight some of the most common and deadly diseases. Research has shown that vitamin E may help prevent or mitigate the effects of chronic diseases such as heart disease, cancer, Alzheimer's disease, and diabetes.

How it helps your heart: Vitamin E has been studied for many years, and there is solid evidence—including double-blind clinical trials—that 400–800 IU of natural vitamin E can reduce heart disease and heart attacks. In fact, several population studies have shown that vitamin E levels may be more predictive of the risk of a heart attack or stroke than even total cholesterol levels. Some studies show that high-cholesterol levels are predictive of a heart attack 29% of the time. High blood pressure was predictive 25% of the time. However, low levels of vitamin E were predictive 70% of the time.[20]

The largest study to date on vitamin E and heart disease was conducted by researchers at Harvard University. It looked at approximately 90,000 nurses and their intake of vitamin E. The results suggested that the incidence of heart disease was 30%–40% lower among nurses with the highest intake of vitamin E from diet and supplements.[21,22] Very similar results were found in approximately 40,000 men in the Health Professionals Follow-up Study. The men who took vitamin-E supplements reduced their risk of heart disease by 37%.[23]

A daily dose of 400–800 IU of natural vitamin E cut subsequent heart attacks in men with heart problems by an astonishing 77%.[24] Other research shows that it takes 400 IU of vitamin E to squelch the oxidation of LDL cholesterol.[25] For more on the importance of oxidation when discussing LDL cholesterol, see "Myth 2" in chapter 7.

An extensive study at the National Institute of Aging of approximately 11,000 seniors found that elderly people who supplemented with Vitamin E had a 41% reduction in heart disease, a 27% lower risk of all-cause mortality, and even a 22% reduction in death from cancer.[26] In another study, vitamin-E users were 47% less apt to die of heart disease and 59% less likely to die of cancer. Taking vitamin E *and* vitamin C in high doses cut chances of death from all causes by 42%.[27]

Safety Concerns of Vitamin E

A recent study published in the *Annals of Internal Medicine* states that high doses of vitamin E (400 IU or more per day) are dangerous. Is that true? If so, does the danger outweigh the benefit of vitamin-E supplements?

Let's investigate the study mentioned. It was an analysis of several studies involving the use of vitamin E for various diseases, but it did not include some observational studies that have shown a correlation between vitamin-E use and a reduced risk of coronary disease. Also, in the studies analyzed, vitamin E was often used in combination with pharmaceutical drugs; the effects of these combinations were not discussed in the analysis. In addition, the populations being studied mostly consisted of elderly people with chronic diseases. The paper recognizes this as a possible negative variable, because elderly, sick people are more likely to be taking high doses of vitamin E. It would not be possible to generalize the findings to a young and healthy population.

The analysis looked at different types of research studies that used different protocols and procedures, such as different doses of vitamin E taken for different lengths of time. The original studies didn't necessarily differentiate between natural and synthetic vitamin E. Therefore, some of the results of the original studies have been subsequently questioned.

The bottom line is that the Institute of Medicine and the federal government agree that vitamin E is safe at levels as high as 1,600 IU per day for *natural* vitamin E (the form I recommend) or 1,000 IU for synthetic vitamin E, the form often used in research studies.

MULTIVITAMINS

The composition and quality of multivitamins is as varied as the colors of the spectrum. So you have to read the labels—not only the ingredients, but the brands. Some truly are better than others and will provide better results.

How they help your heart: Multivitamin use has been shown to reduce mortality rates in general, and heart-disease deaths specifically. One large-scale study examined vitamin use and mortality rates of a million people in the United States. Those who took multivitamins containing vitamins A, C, and E had significantly reduced risk of heart-disease related deaths.[28]

Another study looked at the effect of a multivitamin over the course of a six-month period on adults with stress and/or exhaustion. Participants were given pretest measures of psychological and neurological symptoms. After the six months ended, participants noted an overall 40% reduction in stress, an almost 25% reduction of negative conditions, and an almost 20% increase in positive conditions. There was also 30% fewer infections reported, as well as a 91% decrease in intestinal pain. This suggests that the daily use of an oral multivitamin supplement will help reduce stress and many of the physical symptoms of stress.[29]

B vitamins can actually decrease the amount of plaque in arteries, including carotid (neck) arteries, where a blockage can cause a stroke. In a four-year study, plague in carotid arteries decreased by 10% for those taking 250 mcg. B12, 25 mg. B6, and 2,500 mcg. folic acid (a form of B9). Plaque increased by 50% in the non-vitamin-B takers. (Note: 800 mcg. of folic acid is effective for most people, according to the researchers.)[30]

Dr. Mark Houston, associate clinical professor of medicine at Vanderbilt University and author of *What Your Doctor May Not Tell You About Hypertension,* reports that the medical journals are overflowing with studies (over 1,000 of them) that demonstrate the effectiveness of various supplements and foods in the treatment of hypertension.[31] From my experience, there are just as many studies that validate the benefits of natural nutrients in the treatment of heart disease.

More Benefits of Multivitamins

One research study examined the effect of an oral multivitamin supplement on psychological well-being and functioning. Male participants who were free of chronic medical problems were given either a multivitamin or a placebo during the course of 28 days. (Participants were not aware of which kind of supplement they were taking.) At the conclusion of the study, those participants who had taken the multivitamin reported a significant reduction in anxiety and stress levels. They also reported improved concentration and less fatigue. The patients taking the placebo continued to report body pains, nausea, and headaches—symptoms associated with anxiety—more often than did those taking the multivitamin.[32]

Studies have shown that multivitamins improve IQ levels in children.[33] And in those 65 or older, multivitamins have proven to significantly improve memory, abstract thinking, problem-solving ability, and attention span.[34] Bernard Gesch's double-blind trial on young offenders in a maximum-security prison in Aylesbury really proved how powerful nutrients are on mood and behavior. He gave the inmates either a multinutrient—containing vitamins, minerals, and essential fatty acids—or a placebo. The results, published in the *British Journal of Psychiatry,* showed a staggering 35% decrease in acts of aggression after only two weeks. When the trial was over and the supplements were stopped, there was a 40% increase in offenses in the prison.[35] If multivitamins can do that to Britain's young offenders in two weeks, just think what they could do for the rest of us.

A research study published in the Lancet took a group of 96 healthy, elderly people and gave some a high-potency multivitamin-mineral and others a placebo for a year. Those on the supplements had half the number of "infection days" and a highly significant increase in immune strength as measured by cell counts in blood tests.[36]

Conventional vs. Natural Treatments

I could continue for several hundred pages about the benefits of nutrients. But let's take a look at some specific heart diagnoses you might have received. We'll briefly examine their conventional treatments as well as safe, effective, natural alternatives.

Mitral Valve Prolapse (MVP): Conventional medical treatments for MVP typically involve one of the following beta blockers: Inderal, Lopressor, Tenormin, Toprol, or Blocadren. Beta blockers slow the heart rate by blocking the cell receptors for epinephrine (adrenaline). But by slowing the heart rate, these drugs may increase the pressure placed on the blood vessel lining. This can cause further damage to already damaged or clogged arteries.

Beta blockers have several other potential side effects: congestive heart failure (CHF), shortness of breath, heart block, fatigue, lethargy, drowsiness, depression, insomnia, colitis, headaches, dizziness, tingling in the hands and feet, wheezing, bronchospasm, increased severity of asthma or chronic pulmonary obstructive disease, Raynaud's syndrome (involving burning, tingling, and numbness), decreased sex drive, muscle fatigue, reduced HDL cholesterol, increased LDL cholesterol and triglycerides, and type-2 diabetes.[37]

I've found that most patients can overcome true MVP without the use of prescription beta blockers. But they will need to address the underlying cause(s) of their illness. This involves building up their **natural stress-coping chemicals** and abilities through restoring adequate levels of serotonin, cortisol, DHEA, essential fatty acids, and other vitamins, minerals, and essential nutrients. Many people with MVP have true dysautonomia, a disruption of the autonomic nervous system, which can also lead to fibromyalgia. Many of my fibromyalgia patients (I would estimate 70%) also have MVP. Both fibromyalgia and symptomatic MVP are triggered by acute or chronic stress and result in dysautonomia.

So if you have been diagnosed with MVP, I strongly suggest that you investigate dysautonomia and follow my procedures for battling it as outlined in my first book, *Treating and Beating Fibromyalgia and Chronic Fatigue Syndrome.*

As for using a beta blocker for MVP, I recommend, instead of a dangerous chemical, the natural beta blocker described earlier in this chapter: **magnesium.** It naturally inhibits stimulatory hormones, including norepinephrine and epinephrine. Fortunately magnesium—as a natural substance your body needs anyway—doesn't cause the symptoms associated with prescription beta blockers.

Some studies show that those with MVP are deficient in magnesium.[38] Other studies show that magnesium reduces the symptoms of MVP, including palpitations, chest pain, and fatigue.[39]

Atrial Fibrillation: This is a serious health concern best monitored by your cardiologist. However, there's no reason why you can't help to reduce your symptoms through nutritional therapies that have been shown effective for those with atrial fibrillation.

Conventional therapies for managing atrial fibrillation rely on diuretics, calcium-channel blockers, and ACE-inhibitor medications. For a discussion of these medications, see chapter 2. The best remedy for atrial fibrillation is prevention. The following nutrients have demonstrated their ability to both prevent and help stabilize atrial fibrillation: **Fish oil** (DHA and EPA) increases certain hormones (prostaglandin 1) that help relax heart-muscle spasms.[40] The recommended dose is 4–9 g. a day. **Bromelain,** as a derivative of pineapple, acts as a powerful anti-inflammatory and reduces blood pressure, platelet clumping, fibrinogen levels, and atrial fibrillation.[41] The recommended dose is 750 mg. three times a day on an empty stomach.

Congestive Heart Failure and Other Heart Diseases: Conventional medical therapy for CHF includes diuretics, ACE inhibitors, beta blockers, and calcium-channel blockers. But these medications, while they treat the symptoms, actually accelerate the rate of CHF.[42] When taking diuretics, which cause a magnesium deficiency, a person should at the very least increase their dietary magnesium intake. Even better is to add a good comprehensive multivitamin-mineral supplement with a minimum of 400–600 mg. of **magnesium.** Have I mentioned yet that magnesium is essential for proper heart function?

Well, sorry to bore you, but I'm going to say it again. As more research is completed, magnesium may prove to be the most important nutrient in facilitating optimal cardiovascular health. Studies have already demonstrated that low magnesium levels decrease the survival rate in those with CHF—by almost 50%.[43]

The natural herb **hawthorne** has also been proven in double-blind studies to help reduce the symptoms associated with CHF.[44] The recommended dose is 200 mg. three times a day.

Numerous double-blind studies have demonstrated the importance of **L-carnitine** in the management of CHF. [45,46,47] This amino acid delivers long-chain fatty acids to the heart, and these fatty acids provide 70% of the heart's energy. That's because the mitochondria use them to create ATP, which powers every cell in the body. The heart needs a *lot* of ATP, for obvious reasons, so it is sensitive to even minor deficiencies in ATP-building nutrients like carnitine and CoQ10.

L-carnitine increases heart-muscle productivity while preventing fatty-acid buildup in the heart and liver. It also removes waste products from cells for maximum metabolic efficiency. It can be purchased over-the-counter, and carnitine-replacement therapy has been shown to reduce cardiac arrhythmia and angina. The recommended dose is 500 mg. three times a day on an empty stomach. For those with congestive heart failure or progressive heart disease, I've recommended as much as 4,000 mg. daily, in divided doses.

Arginine, an amino acid, helps dilate (relax and open) blood vessels that have been unresponsive to drug therapy. Studies involving arginine have shown that it acts like the drug nitroglycerine, which increases nitric oxide. Because of its vasodilating abilities, arginine is recommended for the management of angina. It also helps boost blood flow to the extremities (legs) by up to 29%.[48] The recommended dose is 1,000–12,000 mg. a day, preferably on an empty stomach.

As already explained, **CoQ10** has an impressive track record in regards to CHF. But let me throw in a couple more reports about it. In one study, patients were administered a modest 30 mg. of CoQ10 a day. All the participants in the study showed improvement, and 53% were asymptomatic after four weeks.[49] The largest study to date on CoQ10 involved 2,664 patients with congestive heart failure and was conducted in Italy. The results showed that individuals who took an average of 100 mg. of CoQ10 a day for three months noticed a drastic improvement in their symptoms: cyanosis (78% of patients improved), edema (fluid retention) (79%), vertigo (73%), insomnia (66%), sweating (80%), shortness of breath (52%), pulmonary edema (fluid on the lungs) (78%), enlarged liver (49%), heart palpitations (75%), arrhythmia (abnormal heartbeat) (63%), venous congestion (72%).[50]

D-ribose is a naturally occurring sugar, a component of RNA, and a critical component for all your cells. It's used by the body to make ATP and other essential chemicals. Ischemic heart disease (IHD) may cause the heart to lose up to 50% of its ATP supply, so anyone with IHD will want to do whatever he can to increase his ATP levels. D-ribose is the *only* compound used by the human body to restore diminished ATP stores. By restoring ATP levels, D-ribose increases cardiac function and energy. It can restore diastolic blood pressure to normal within days of beginning replacement therapy.

Patients with heart failure or progressive IHD will benefit the most from taking D-ribose (I would recommend 10–15 g. daily). However, it's also an excellent supplement for preventing disease, especially if you have any signs of early heart disease, have high blood pressure, or are taking statin drugs. In this case, I would recommend at least 5 g. daily. D-ribose, though a sugar, doesn't raise blood-sugar levels in most people. Even type-2 diabetics will likely be able to take it without concern. As with any sugar, type-1 diabetics should monitor their levels closely to learn how D-ribose affects them.

Another great recommendation I have for those with heart disease is the book *Reverse Heart Disease Now*[51] by two medical doctors, Sinatra and Roberts. They offer a thorough discussion of CoQ10, L-carnitine, and D-ribose in their relation to heart disease.

Natural Versions of Cardiac Drugs

Here's a reference list (with thanks to Mark Houston[52]) of natural alternatives to drugs normally prescribed for heart conditions.

- **Natural calcium-channel blockers** include magnesium, alpha lipoic acid, hawthorne berry, vitamin B6, omega-3 fatty acids, and garlic.
- **A natural beta blocker** is hawthorne berry. You can take 100–250 mg. of standardized (10% procyanidins) hawthorne-berry extract three times a day.
- **Supplements that act like ACE-II drugs** include vitamin B6, vitamin C, garlic, and potassium.
- **Natural vasodilators** include omega-3 fatty acids, garlic, celery, L-arginine, and taurine.

Treating Heart Disease with Supplements

- Everyone should be taking a good optimal-daily-allowance multivitamin-mineral supplement with a minimum of 400 mg. of magnesium daily. Take this with food.
- Take a minimum of 2,000 mg. of fish oil a day, also with food.
- If you have a heart condition or high blood pressure, take 100–200 mg. of CoQ10 a day.
- If you have CHF, take a minimum 500 mg. of L-carnitine three times a day on an empty stomach.
- For chronic chest pain, consider L-arginine.
- Consider supplementing with a special formula called Cardio-Stolix (you read about this at the end of chapter 6) or my Healthy Heart Formula, which contains an optimal daily multivitamin-mineral with 500 mg. of magnesium, 100 mg. of CoQ10, 2,000 mg. of fish oil, and odorless garlic extract. (See the appendix for ordering information.)
- Those with CHF or other diseased-heart conditions should consider supplementing with D-ribose and L-carnitine as directed above.

Notes

1. Mark C. Houston, Barry Fox, and Nadine Taylor, *What Your Doctor May Not Tell You About Hypertension: The Revolutionary Nutrition and Lifestyle Program to Help Fight High Blood Pressure* (New York: Grand Central, 2003).
2. Roberto Marchioli, et al., "Early Protection Against Sudden Death by n-3 Polyunsaturated Fatty Acids After Myocardial Infarction," *Circulation* 105 (2002): 1897.
3. Claude A. Allen (Deputy Secretary), Department of Health and Human Services, Executive Office of the President, Office of Management and Budget, "To Save Lives, OMB Urges Revising Dietary Guidelines" (May 28, 2003).
4. S.H. Jee et al., "The Effect of Magnesium Supplementation on Blood Pressure: a Meta-analysis of Randomized Clinical Trials," *American Journal of Hypertension* 15 (2002): 691–6.
5. F.J. Simoes et al., "Therapeutic Effect of a Magnesium Salt in Patients Suffering from Mitral Valvular Prolapse and Latent Tetany," *Magnesium* 4(5–6) (1985): 283–90.
6. M. Shechter et al., "Oral Magnesium Therapy Improves Endothelial Function in Patients with Coronary Artery Disease," *Circulation* 102(19) (2000): 2353–8.
7. H. Yasue and K. Kugiyama, "Spasm: Clinical Features and Pathogenesis," *Kumamoto University School of Medicine* 36(11) (1997): 760–5.
8. Sandy Simmons, "Mitral Valve Prolapse: What Causes It? Can Diet Changes Help?" *Sandy Simmons's Connective Tissue Disorder Site,* web article, www.ctds.info/mvp1.html#mitral_valve_prolapse, referencing *Scandinavian Journal of Clinical and Laboratory Investigation* (supplement) 224 (1996): 211–34.
9. ibid.
10. B.M. Altura and B.T. Altura, "New Perspectives on the Role of Magnesium in the Pathophysiology of the Cardiovascular System," *Magnesium* 4(5–6) (1985).
11. N.M. Ramadan et al., "Low Brain Magnesium in Migraine Headache," *Journal of Head and Face Pain* 29(7) (2005): 416–9.
12. Rodger Murphree, *Treating and Beating Fibromyalgia and Chronic Fatigue Syndrome* (Birmingham: Harrison and Hampton, 2003).
13. T. Oda et al., "Stress Echocardiography for Pediatric Patients with Symptomatic Mitral Valve Prolapse," *Japanese Circulation Journal* 47 (1983): 1335.
14. Emile G. Bliznakov and Gerald L. Hunt, The *Miracle Nutrient Coenzyme Q10* (New York: Bantan, 1986).
15. Peter H. Langsjoen, "Introduction to Coenzyme Q10," University of Washington, http://faculty.washington.edu/ely/coenzq10.html.
16. W.V. Judy et al., "Coenzyme Q10 Reduction of Adrianmycin Cardiotoxicity," *Biomedical and Clinical Aspects of Coenzyme Q10* 4 (Elsevier Science, 1984): 231–41.
17. ibid.
18. P. Langjoen, R. Willis, and K. Folkers, "Treatment of Essential Hypertension with Coenzyme Q10," *Molecular Aspects of Medicine* 15 (1994): S265–72.

19. Stephen Sinatra, *The CoQ10 Phenomenon* (Chicago: Keats, 1998), 54.
20. M.C. Bellizzi, M.F. Franklin, and G.G. Duthie, "Vitamin E and Coronary Heart Disease: the European Paradox," *European Journal of Clinical Nutrition* 48 (1994): 822–31.
21. Eric B. Rimm et al., "Vitamin E Consumption and the Risk of Coronary Heart Disease in Men," *New England Journal of Medicine* 328 (1993): 1450–6.
22. Meir J. Stampfer et al., "Vitamin E Consumption and the Risk of Coronary Disease in Women," *New England Journal of Medicine* 328 (1993): 1444–9.
23. Eric B. Rimm et al., "Vitamin E Consumption and the Risk of Coronary Heart Disease in Men," *New England Journal of Medicine* 328 (1993): 1450–6.
24. ibid.
25. L. Jialal and S. Grundy, "Effect of Dietary Supplementation with Alpha-tocopherol on the Oxidative Modification of Low Density Lipoprotein," *Journal of Lipid Research* 33 (1992): 899–906.
26. K.G. Losonczy et al., "Vitamin E and Vitamin C Supplement Use and Risk of All-cause and Coronary Heart Disease Mortality in Older Persons: The Established Populations for Epidemiologic Studies of the Elderly," *American Journal of Clinical Nutrition* 64 (1996): 190–6.
27. ibid.
28. M.L. Watkins et al., "Multivitamin Use and Mortality in a Large Prospective Study," *American Journal of Epidemiology* 152(2) (2000): 149–62.
29. J. Gruenwald, H.J. Graubaum, and A. Harde, "Effect of a Probiotic Multi-vitamin Compound on Stress and Exhaustion," *Advances in Therapy* 19(3) (2002): 141-50.
30. BioInfoBank Library, "Hyperhomocysteinemia: Complications," http://lib.bioinfo.pl/meid:48784.
31. Mark Houston, *What Your Doctor May Not Tell You About Hypertension* (New York: Time Warner, 2003).
32. D. Carroll, et al., "The Effects of an Oral Multivitamin Combination with Calcium, Magnesium, and Zinc on Psychological Well-being in Healthy Young Male Volunteers: a Double-blind Placebo-controlled Trial," *Psychopharmacology* 150(2) (2000): 220–5.
33. "Natural Mind and Memory Boosters," Family Education, web article, http://life.familyeducation.com/mental-health/social-emotional/35987.html?page=6.
34. R.K. Chandra, "Effect of Vitamin and Trace-element Supplementation on Cognitive Function in Elderly Subjects," *Nutrition* 17(9) (2001): 709–12.
35. B. Gesch, "Influence of Supplementary Vitamins, Minerals and Essential Fatty Acids on the Antisocial Behavior of Young Adult Prisoners," *British Journal of Psychiatry* 181 (2002): 22–8.
36. R.K. Chandra, "Study of Multivitamin/mineral Supplementation in Elderly," *Lancet* 340: 1124–7.

37. Mark C. Houston, Barry Fox, and Nadine Taylor, *What Your Doctor May Not Tell You About Hypertension: The Revolutionary Nutrition and Lifestyle Program to Help Fight High Blood Pressure* (New York: Grand Central, 2003).
38. F.J. Simoes et al., "Therapeutic Effect of a Magnesium Salt in Patients Suffering from Mitral Valvular Prolapse and Latent Tetany," *Magnesium* 4(5–6) (1985): 283–90.
39. M. Shechter et al., "Oral Magnesium Therapy Improves Endothelial Function in Patients with Coronary Artery Disease," *Circulation* 7;102(19) (2000): 2353–8.
40. J. Braly, *Dr. Braly's Optimum Health Program* (New York: Times, 1989).
41. J.A. Duke, *The Green Pharmacy* (New York: St. Martins, 2002).
42. Milton Packer, Stephen S. Gottlieb, and Paul D. Kessler, "Hormone-Electrolyte Interactions in the Pathogenesis of Lethal Cardiac Arrhythmias in Patients with Congestive Heart Failure," *American Journal of Medicine* 80 (supplement 4a) (1986): 23–9.
43. S.S. Gottlieb et al., "Prognostic Importance of Serum Magnesium Concentration in Patients with Congestive Heart Failure," *Journal of the American College of Cardiology* 16 (1990): 827–31.
44. M. O'Conolly, W. Jansen, and G. Bernhoft, "Treatment of Decreasing Performance: Therapy Using Standardized Crataegus Extract in Advanced Age," *Fortschritte der Medizin* 104 (1986): 805–8.
45. R. Crayhon, *The Carnitine Miracle* (Manhattan: M. Evans and Company, 1998).
46. L. Cacciatore et al., "The Therapeutic Effect of L-Carnitine in Patients with Exercise-induced Stable Angina: a Controlled Study," *Drugs Under Experimental and Clinical Research* 17(4) (1991): 225–35.
47. P. Pola, "Statistical Evaluation of Long-term L-Carnitine Therapy in Hyperlipoproteinemias," *Drugs Under Experimental and Clinical Research* 9 (1983): 925–34.
48. T.S. Rector et al., "Randomized, Double-blind, Placebo-controlled Study of Supplemental Oral L-Arginine in Patients with Heart Failure," *Circulation* 93(12) (1996): 2135–41.
49. T. Ishiyama et al., "A Clinical Study of the Effect of Coenzyme Q10 on Congestive Heart Failure," *Japanese Heart Journal* 17 (1976): 32.
50. E. Baggio, R. Gandini, and A.C. Plancher, "Italien Multicenter Study on the Safety and Efficacy of Coenzyme Q10 as an Adjunctive Therapy in Heart Failure," *Molecular Aspects of Medicine* 15 (1994): s287–94.
51. Stephen T. Sinatra and James C. Roberts, *Reverse Heart Disease Now: Stop Deadly Cardiovascular Plaque Before It's Too Late* (Hoboken: John Wiley & Sons, 2007).
52. Mark C. Houston, Barry Fox, and Nadine Taylor, *What Your Doctor May Not Tell You About Hypertension: The Revolutionary Nutrition and Lifestyle Program to Help Fight High Blood Pressure* (New York: Grand Central, 2003).

10

What *Really* Causes Heart Disease?

FOR DECADES, DOCTORS HAVE VIEWED HEART DISEASE in terms of plaque buildup and clogged arteries. Cholesterol and triglycerides were the villains. The theory was that after years of poor diet, fatty deposits or plaques would start to build up within the arteries. Eventually, this plaque would grow so large that it would cut off the blood supply to the heart, resulting in angina, high blood pressure, and—for those not treated with cholesterol-lowering drugs—a heart attack. Studies that showed a correlation between cholesterol levels and heart disease fueled the flames of panic.

As concern grew, doctors militantly advocated that cholesterol levels be below 200 (this number has steadily dropped over the years). A campaign was waged to educate the public about the differences between LDL and HDL cholesterol, labeling one "bad," and the other "good." All the public knew was that a high LDL and a low HDL spelled trouble, so they rushed to attack their levels with lipid-lowering drugs, especially statins.

There were, however, some serious problems with this script. Half of all heart attacks were occurring in people with *normal* cholesterol levels! And surprisingly, diagnostic imaging showed that the most dangerous plaques were actually not very large. In fact, half of all those with coronary artery disease didn't have *any* of the traditional risk factors.[1] Clearly there were other factors involved.

Dozens of theories attempt to explain the cause of atherosclerosis, arteriosclerosis, and heart disease. Scientific studies have documented the ill effects of total cholesterol, elevated LDL, low HDL, homocysteines, fibrinogen, oxidative stress, elevated c-reactive protein levels, inflammation, sedentary lifestyles, diabetes, obesity, infections, and stress.

What We Do Know

The endothelial lining of the artery becomes damaged from physical, chemical, viral, bacterial, or immune reactions. Once damaged, it becomes more permeable to lipoproteins (fat-carrying proteins), and the arterial lining's connective tissue begins to deteriorate, attracting cholesterol deposits. Large white blood cells (monocytes) and blood-clotting platelets attach themselves to the injured area, causing plaque to form. A fibrous cap (consisting of collagen, elastin, and glycosaminoglycans) forms over the injured area.

Cholesterol and fat begin to build up around the site, and an arthroma is formed. The arthroma, made of fibrous-coated plaque, may continue to grow until it eventually blocks the flow of blood through the artery. It usually takes a 90% blockage to experience any symptoms of atherosclerosis. Arthromas may calcify, hardening in a process known as arteriosclerosis. Atherosclerosis of the coronary arteries may lead to thrombosis (blood clot formation), which manifests itself as angina (chest pain) or a heart attack. Atherosclerosis of the cerebral (brain) arteries can trigger a stroke.

As you can see, cholesterol is not the cause of arteriosclerosis. Like white blood cells, it is part of the injury-repair process. If we are going to wipe out cholesterol, why not just wipe out the white blood cells? Of course this is a silly question; we all know how important WBCs are to our very survival. Cholesterol plays *just* as vital a role in regulating various bodily functions. Attacking cholesterol with prescription medications ignores the real question: What is the cause of the inflammation that leads to the damage, and how do we reduce it? The information below gets a little complicated. But hang in there; this is important.

Inflammation in Detail

Numerous bodily interactions can trigger inflammation, which then leads to cellular damage. Certain inflammatory chemicals are manufactured from the foods (principally fats) we eat. Too much omega-6, for instance, can create inflammation. Trauma, infection, ischemia (reduced blood flow), toxins, poisons, and normal wear-and-tear can also cause an inflammatory response by the body's self-regulating mechanisms.

When inflammation leads to blood-vessel damage, the vessels dilate (expand). This dilation causes the area to become hot, red, and swollen. Then the debris from the cell damage must be disposed of. Inflammatory prostaglandins (PG-2) trigger the WBCs to come help clean up the cellular mess, attacking and digesting damaged cells and tissues. As their work is completed, the healthy tissue surrounding the damaged area releases anti-inflammatory prostaglandins (PG-1 and PG-3) to combat the PG-2s. Then proteolytic enzymes are responsible for telling the WBCs that their job is done. They sound the "all clear." As the damaged cells and tissues are removed, less of the pro-inflammatory chemicals and more of the anti-inflammatory chemicals are released. Once the inflammation process is finished, the body begins to repair itself as described above.

The balance between inflammation, destruction, and repair is an ongoing process that is normally kept in check. But when the process becomes unbalanced, chronic inflammation takes over.

Inflammation is largely regulated by the prostaglandin hormones. If we can help these hormones do their job by not overworking them, then our bodies can age gracefully, regulating their own inflammatory processes and repairing damage only as needed. This is the principle behind the inflammation theory of heart disease. It is a theory to which I heartily subscribe. But before I talk about specific ways to reduce inflammation in the body, it's time for a little vocabulary lesson.

Types of Fats

You often hear the terms *fat* and *lipid* used interchangeably. Lipids are substances that can't be dissolved in water and include fats, oils, and phospholipids (lecithin). Fat is made up of fatty acids. There are three main types of fatty acids.

Saturated fatty acids (SFAs) are found in butter, coconut oil, eggs, meat, and cheese. Saturated fats consist of long, straight chains of molecules packed tightly together. They are solid at room temperature.

Monounsaturated fatty acids (MUFAs) are found in almond oil, avocados, canola oil, oats, peanut oil, and olive oil. Monounsaturated oils are usually liquid at room temperature and may become cloudy or hardened when placed in the refrigerator. MUFAs have one bend in their chain structure, and this makes them more flexible than SFAs.

Polyunsaturated fatty acids (PUFAs) are found in oils from cold-water fish, corn, primrose, flaxseed, borage, sesame, sunflower, safflower, and wheat germ. Vegetable cooking oils are usually high in PUFAs, which are liquid at room temperature. PUFAs have many bends in their fatty-acid chains, so they are soft and flexible. Polyunsaturated fatty acids are how we get the essential fatty acids, omega-3 and omega-6.

Essential Fatty Acids

Essential fatty acids are fats that can't be made by the body; they must be obtained from the foods we eat. There are two types.

Omega-6 (linoleic acid) is found in pure vegetable oils, including sunflower, safflower, and corn oil.

Omega-3 (linolenic acid) is found in flax seed, soybean, walnut, and chestnut oils, as well as some dark-green, leafy vegetables. Certain omega-3 foods, including cold-water fish, also contain eicosapentaenoic acid (EPA) and docosahexanoic acid (DHA). EPA plays an important role in reducing inflammation.

It is the essential fatty acids that create the prostaglandins.

Prostaglandins and Inflammation

There are over 30 different prostaglandins. (Although prostaglandins are found throughout the body, they're named for the sheep gland in which they were first discovered—the prostate.) Remember that prostaglandins are the hormones that regulate the inflammation process. The PG-2 hormone *causes* inflammation; PG-1 and PG-3 *reduce* inflammation.

Omega-6 is responsible for creating PG-1 and PG-2. Omega-3 creates PG-3.

Arachidonic Acid and PG-2

The pro-inflammatory hormone PG-2 is made (by omega-6) from a substance called arachidonic acid (AA).

AA initiates platelet aggregation (blood clotting) and increases salt reuptake by the kidneys, which can lead to swelling and an increase in blood pressure. It stimulates the production of inflammatory chemicals, including leukotriens (notorious for causing allergic reactions), thromboxanes, and prostacylins.

AA is found in corn, safflower, and other vegetable oils. Though AA wouldn't naturally be found at high levels in meat, corn products are used as the prominent foodstuff in westernized livestock, and this creates meat and dairy products with a high-AA content. Several research articles have demonstrated that the more animal fats a human eats, the more AA she has in her blood and her cell membranes. This makes her more likely to become inflamed. Vegetable oils used to manufacture processed foods are the greatest source of AA, so eating processed foods also increases AA levels in the body.

Fish Oils and PG-3

Conversely, a diet high in fish oils promotes *less* inflammation and a *lower* level of inflammatory chemicals. This occurs because omega-3 not only produces the anti-inflammatory PG-3 but also helps prevent omega-6 from turning into AA. It's interesting to note that hunter-gatherer societies had a 1:1 to 1:5 ratio of omega-6 to omega-3. Modern eating habits have changed this to a 12:1 ratio. We are eating way too much omega-6. And 60% percent of the U.S. population is deficient in omega-3.[2]

The healthiest ratio (about 1.5:1) is found in Japanese populations, which also have the highest life expectancy and the lowest rate of cardiovascular disease. Go figure! There's no way around the fact that our inflammatory reactions and their chemicals are largely determined by what foods (fatty acids) we eat.[3]

Since most Americans are carrying around 10–20 pounds of excess fat (the majority of which is AA), it is no wonder that arteriosclerosis, arthritis, and other inflammatory diseases are out of control in our country! An increase in omega-6 results in an increased risk of rheumatoid and other inflammatory-related illnesses.[4]

Reducing Heart Disease by Reducing Inflammation

When it comes to heart disease, your food choices could literally save your life. So consider your heart when you eat.

Limit meat, dairy, and vegetable oils. Since vegetable oils, seed oils, and corn-fed livestock have high AA levels, I suggest patients reduce products from these sources. Choose milk and meat from free-range, grass-fed livestock whenever possible. Cook with canola oil, peanut oil, or olive oil.

Increase fish oils. Increasing omega-3 fish oils lowers blood pressure, reduces blood clotting, helps normalize heart arrhythmias, and decreases the risk of stroke and heart attack. Some studies have shown that supplementing with fish oils results in a dramatic reduction in a person's leukotriens (one of the chemicals implicated in asthma and other allergic reactions) by 65%. This correlates with a 75% decrease in their clinical symptoms.[5] Another fish-oil study involved rheumatoid arthritis sufferers (often treated with incredibly toxic and life-threatening prescription drugs) who took 1.8 grams of EPA fish oil and reduced their land-animal foods. These patients showed significant improvement over and above those treated with a placebo.[6,7]

So consume at least two servings of cold-water fish a week or take fish-oil supplements as described in chapter 6. Those with heart disease should consume 2–6 g. of fish oil a day. Those with arthritis or other inflammatory diseases may need to take up to 9 g. a day for 2–3 months before they notice a difference in their symptoms.

Avoid trans fats. Obtaining essential fatty acids from the foods we eat can be challenging, since much of our foods has undergone processing that changes them into hydrogenated oils, creating toxic trans fatty acids. If you have heart disease, high blood pressure, or an inflammation-related disease like arthritis, colitis, or allergies, then you'll need to reduce your consumption of polyunsaturated foods. But everyone should avoid trans fatty acids.

Keep a healthy weight. Pro-inflammatory PG-2 is stored in fat. So if you are overweight, here's another good reason to shed those extra pounds.

We are what we eat. We've heard this before, but perhaps have never really thought about its true ramifications. We can positively alter our health by changing our diet. But first we must separate fact from fiction. In chapter 12, we'll look at some diet *myths.* But first let's investigate some new, more reliable markers for heart disease.

Notes

1. A.R. Gaby, Editorial, *Townsend Letter for Doctors* (August/September 1991): 675.
2. Leo Galland, "Leaky Gut Syndromes: Breaking the Vicious Cycle," The Third International Symposium on Functional Medicine, Vancouver (1996).
3. Andrew Stoll, *The Omega-3 Connection* (New York: Fireside, 2001).
4. ibid.
5. W.F. Stevenson, et al., "Dietary Supplementation with Fish Oil in Ulcerative Colitis," *Annals of Internal Medicine* 11 (1992): 609–14.
6. J. Kremer et al., "Effects of Manipulation of Dietary Fatty Acids on Clinical Manifestation of Rheumatoid Arthritis," *Lancet* (1985): 184–7.
7. J. Kremer, "N-3 Fatty Acid Supplements in Rheumatoid Arthritis," *American Journal of Clinical Nutrition* 71(supplement) (2000): 349–51.

11

Reliable Markers for Heart Disease

WHILE A GREAT DEAL OF TIME, MONEY, AND RESOURCES have gone into the nationwide campaign to prove that cholesterol causes heart disease, newer, more reliable markers for the illness are now available.

FREE RADICALS

Free radicals are unstable atoms or molecules that have an unpaired electron in their outer ring. They react by taking an electron from another molecule, and that molecule then becomes unstable. This sets up a destructive cycle that can damage tissue.

Free radicals can form naturally in our bodies through internal metabolic activities, including immune and detoxification processes. External sources of free-radical production include radiation, alcohol, tobacco, smog, medications, and pesticides. Believe it or not, though, *oxygen* is responsible for most of the toxic free radicals. Just like the rust on a car, excessive oxygenation to the body can cause premature aging and dysfunction, leading to such conditions as heart disease, rheumatoid arthritis, Alzheimer's, Parkinson's, and cancer.[1,2] Have you ever cut open an apple and then left it out for awhile? If so, then you've witnessed oxygenation and free-radical damage. The once white, inner meat of the apple turns brown when exposed to oxygen. Sprinkling lemon juice on the apple will turn the brown back to its normal color. This is an example of an antioxidant at work.

Inside the body, free radicals can damage cell membranes by interacting with low-density lipoproteins to form lipid peroxides. Lipid peroxides, or damaged fats, cause cholesterol to become oxidized, leading to arteriosclerosis.

How to Battle Them: The good news is that we don't have to just let free radicals have their way. Antioxidants help deter the effects of free-radical damage. These include vitamins A, E, and C; beta carotene; and the amino acids cysteine, methionine, glycine, glutathione,[3] and…brace yourself: *cholesterol.* That's right. Cholesterol is one of the body's most potent antioxidants. It actually protects cell membranes by acting as the body's bounty hunter, scavenging for free radicals on a rampage. Some of the cholesterol-steroid hormones, such as testosterone, dehydroepiandrosterone (DHEA), progesterone, and estrogen can function as antioxidants.[4]

Because cholesterol battles free radicals, levels of cholesterol in your blood will likely increase with an increase of damaging free radicals. In that way, total cholesterol levels might be linked to heart disease…but that doesn't mean that they are the cause of it. It might be that your body is fighting the free radicals (which are leading to the heart disease) by increasing blood levels of cholesterol.

Once cholesterol encounters the free radicals, it can become damaged itself, through oxidation. Oxidized cholesterol, in turn, can damage blood-vessel walls and result in arteriosclerosis.[5]

So in order to reduce the damage caused by free radicals, we must have adequate antioxidants in our system. Low antioxidant status is more predictive of increased risk of heart disease than are cholesterol levels. For instance, a European study found that a low blood level of vitamin E (a potent antioxidant) is 100 times more significant as a risk factor for CAD than is cholesterol.[6]

To raise our levels of antioxidants, we have to consume them. A diet high in fruits and vegetables in combination with a good multivitamin/mineral supplement is all you should need for prevention of free-radical damage.

For individuals with advanced CAD, I recommend supplementing with extra antioxidants such as vitamin C or an extract containing proanthocyanidins (PCOs). These plant-based, free-radical-fighting flavonoids are found in red wine, grape seed, and the bark of the maritime pine. Taking grape-seed extract or pine-bark extracts, then, helps prevent the oxidation of cholesterol and platelet aggregation.[7]

Homocysteine

Homocysteine is a by-product of the conversion of the amino acid cysteine into methionine. If the homocysteine itself is not converted, it will become oxidized by free radicals start to accumulate in the endothelial cells of the arterial wall. This leads to plaque formation and possible arterial occlusion. Homocysteine speeds up the oxidation of cholesterol, which then becomes bound to small LDL particles. White blood cells then infiltrate the particles and transform them into plaque. This plaque begins to grow within the arterial lining, cholesterol swimming through the blood stream attempts to patch the damaged lining, and more plaque occurs.

This entire destructive process begins with too much homocysteine in the blood.

Dr. Kilmer McCully first suggested almost 40 years ago that elevated levels of homocysteine were associated with an increased risk of CAD. He based his theory on autopsies that he and other pathologists conducted on children with a genetic disease called homocystinuria (too much homocysteine) who also had advanced coronary artery disease. Dr. McCully was brazen enough to suggest that cholesterol wasn't promoting arteriosclerosis; the toxic by-product known as homocysteine was.

His theory didn't sit well with his peers at Harvard Medical School, and he was asked to leave. (Unfortunately, Dr. McCully's experience of being ostracized for thinking outside the box is all too common in traditional medicine.) Now, almost 40 years later, his theory has become accepted by all but the most obstinate doctors, as numerous studies have validated his ideas. The *European Journal of Medicine* reported that 40% of those who had strokes also had elevated homocysteine levels, compared to only 6% of controls.[8]

A Norwegian study involving over 4,700 men and women showed that each 5-millimol./l. increase in homocysteine blood plasma caused the number of deaths from all sources to jump 49%. This included a 50% increase in cardiovascular deaths and a 26% increase in cancer deaths.[9]

Based on random hospital blood tests, the prevalence of elevated homocysteine in the elderly with chronic illnesses is estimated at 60%–70%. Seventy percent of those with vascular disease had elevated homocysteine levels, and 63% of those with cognitive dysfunction had elevated homocysteine levels.[10]

How to Battle It: Homocysteine levels should be kept below 7 micromol./l. of blood plasma. Laboratories generally advocate that homocysteine levels are normal up to 15. However, the risk of heart attack goes up greatly when homocysteine levels rise above 6.3 points.[11]

Elevated homocysteine levels are best treated with vitamin B6, vitamin B12, and folic acid. These allow the toxic homocysteine to be converted into its proper end product, cysteine. It is estimated that supplementing with 400 mcg. of folic acid would reduce the number of heart attacks in the United States by 10% (100,000 people) each year.[12] Some individuals with stubborn homocysteine levels will need to add trimethylglycine (TMG) to their supplement therapy.

If you have elevated homocysteine levels, supplement with 500–800 mcg. of folic acid; 1,000–3,000 mcg. of B12; 100–250 mg. of B6; and if needed, 500–900 mg. of TMG (also known as betaine).

By the way, here is what the May 2004 edition of *Harvard Men's Health Watch* had to say about homocysteine: "It's important to maintain a daily intake of 400 micrograms of folic acid and 1.7 milligrams of vitamin B6 if you are over the age of 50. These two vitamins help reduce blood levels of the amino acid homocysteine, now recognized as a risk factor for heart disease and stroke."[13]

Higher levels of homocysteine have also been shown to increase the incidence of deep vein thrombosis.[14] And since homocysteine plays a major role in the metabolism of sulfur and methyl groups, elevated levels most likely impair the synthesis of important nutrients, including SAMe, carnitine, chondroitin sulfate, CoQ10, cysteine, pantetheine, melatonin, phosphatidylcholine, and many others. The resulting deficiency in these nutrients could lead to depression, decreased mental clarity, fatigue, heart disease, increased muscle pain, hypertension, and chemical sensitivities.

C-Reactive Protein

C-Reactive protein (CRP) is manufactured in the liver in response to tissue inflammation and infection. About 20 years ago, two British scientists suggested that CRP was a marker for cardiac injury. As testing procedures became more advanced, their original theory about CRP and heart disease was validated.

A study reported in the *New England Journal Medicine* found that CRP is a *strong* predictor of heart attack and stroke—certainly more predictive than high cholesterol. Men with the highest percentage points had three times the risk of heart attack and twice the risk for stroke.[15] Stroke patients with the highest CRP levels were 2.4 times more likely to die within the next 12 months compared to individuals with the lowest levels of CRP.[16] An elevated CRP level triples your risk of heart attack, even if your LDL cholesterol levels are *normal.*[17] Elevated CRP may indicate inflammation and subsequent arterial-wall damage (which you understand by now results in arteriosclerosis). Certain factors elevate CRP levels, including estrogen-replacement therapy, smoking, type-2 diabetes, a sedentary lifestyle, and infections.

Conventional doctors will often recommend NSAIDs and/or statin drugs to reduce elevated CRP levels. I've already reported the dangers of using NSAIDs for an extended period of time; each year, 10,000–20,000 deaths occur from gastric bleeding. Vioxx and Bextra contributed to thousands of heart-attack deaths.

How to Battle It: You can help keep CRP levels in check by taking vitamin C and other natural anti-inflammatory supplements. (Vitamin C works to lower not only C-reactive protein levels, but blood pressure, fibrinogen levels, and Lp(a) levels.)[18,19] A 10-year study revealed that the more than 11,000 individuals who had high levels of vitamin C extended their lifespan and reduced mortality from cardiovascular disease by 45%.[20] The recommended dose for vitamin C is 2–6 grams a day.

If you already have elevated CRP levels, more aggressive treatment can help.

Fish oil certainly qualifies as a potent anti-inflammatory, as do many of the antioxidants discussed earlier. Vitamin E lowers several inflammation markers, including CRP (by up to 65%).[21] And a rather unconventional but wonderfully useful approach is to supplement your diet with red yeast rice.

Red yeast rice is steamed white rice cultivated with the mold *Monascus purpureus,* which has often been used as a food colorant. Information that led to the creation of statin drugs was harnessed from this rice, sold in jars in Asian markets for years. As it turns out, when the white rice is fermented in this way, chemical are created that block the liver enzyme responsible for producing cholesterol—the same way that statin drugs do artificially. Natural red yeast rice lowers total cholesterol, LDL, and CRP levels without dangerous side effects. It also raises HDL.[22,23] Other natural anti-inflammatories include nattokinase (read about it in chapter 6) and wobezym. Developed in Germany, wobezym has been used by over 100 million people worldwide for 30 years, and it's been shown to reduce CRP levels by a whopping 300%.[24,25]

I personally use an herbal anti-inflammatory formula known (oddly enough) as Inflammation Formula. This product may be available from your naturally oriented health-care professional or from resources listed in the appendix. It contains the following:

- **Tumeric root extract** inhibits enzymes associated with arachidonic acid (PG-2) inflammatory hormones ("the bad guys"—see more about them in chapter 10).
- **Rosemary leaf extract** helps block the synthesis of leukotriens (a cause of allergic inflammation) and prostaglandin 2. It also stimulates phase-II liver detoxification.
- **Holy basil leaf extract** helps boost natural anti-inflammatory chemicals (PG-1 and PG-3).
- **Green tea leaf extract** is a potent antioxidant that increases the body's own anti-inflammatory activity.
- **Ginger root extract** reduces inflammation and helps regulate inflammatory systems.
- **Chinese goldenthread root** helps regulate prostaglandins. It

reduces the activity of the "bad guys" and boosts the function of the "good guys."

- **Barberry root extract** helps regulate prostaglandins, too.
- **Baikal skullcap root extract** reduces inflammatory chemicals, including PG-2.
- **Protykin polygonum cuspidatum extract** is a potent antioxidant that also reduces inflammatory chemicals, including PG-2.

FIBRINOGEN

Another relatively new risk marker for CAD is fibrinogen, a protein involved in blood clotting and platelet clumping. It is increased by inflammation, oxidative damage, smoking, stress, oral contraceptives, and aging. Elevated fibrinogen levels have been shown to increase the incidence of stroke.[26] Increased fibrinogen levels may also cause blood to clot and plaques to form within arterial walls.[27]

The New England Journal of Medicine reports that those with elevated levels of fibrinogen were more than twice as likely as others to die of a heart attack.[28] Research shows that it is best to keep fibrinogen levels below 300 mg/dl.

How to Battle It: Vitamin C is doses of 2,000 mg. or more helps lower fibrinogen.[29]

Garlic acts as a natural blood thinner, so increase your intake if your fibrinogen levels are high. Thinning the blood a bit helps prevent the clotting associated with excess fibrinogen levels.[30] Recommended dose is 4,000 mcg. a day.

Fish-oil supplementation also helps to reduce fibrinogen levels.[31] The recommended dose is 4–9 g. a day. Cod-liver oil also lowers fibrinogen levels.[32]

Curcumin, the yellow pigment found in tumeric, is a powerful antioxidant and a potent anti-inflammatory. Its ability to reduce inflammation helps squelch excess fibrinogen levels.[33]

Ginkgo Biloba has over 300 clinical trials that support its use in the management of cardiovascular and cognitive disorders. It acts as a vasodilator to lower blood pressure, improve blood flow to the extremities (legs), and reduces fibrinogen levels. One study showed that 40 mg. of ginkgo taken twice a day reduced the symptoms associated with intermittent claudication (decreased circulation to the legs) up to 45%.[34] Recommended dose is 80–120 mg. a day.

Vitamin E has been shown to lower fibrinogen levels by as much as 24%.[35]

Notes

1. C.E. Cross et al., "Oxygen Radicals and Human Disease," *Annals of Internal Medicine* 107 (1987): 526–45.
2. P.A. Cerutti, "Oxy-Radicals and Cancer," *Lancet* 344 (1994): 862–3.
3. J.D. Butterfield and C.P. McGraw," Free Radical Pathology," *Stroke* 9(5) (1978): 443–5.
4. W.A. Pryor, "Free Radical Reactions and Their Importance in Biochemical Systems," *Federation Proceedings* 32 (1973):1862–9.
5. Elmer M. Cranton, *Bypassing Bypass Surgery* (Yelm, WA: Medex, 2001), 270.
6. K.F. Gey et al., "Inverse Correlation Between Plasma Vitamin E and Mortality From Ischemic Heart Disease in Cross-cultural Epidemiology," *American Journal of Clinical Nutrition* 53 (1991): 326S–34S.
7. W.C. Chang, "Inhibition of Platelet Aggregation and Arachidonate Metabolism in Platelets by Proancyanidins," *Prostaglandins Leukotrienes and Essential Fatty Acids* 38 (1989): 181–8.
8. L. Brattstrom et al., "Hyperhomocysteinaemia in Stroke: Prevalence, Cause, and Relationships to Type of Stroke and Stroke Risk Factors," *European Journal of Clinical Investigation* 22(3) (1992): 214–21.
9. S.E. Vollset et al., "Plasma Total Homocysteine, Pregnancy Complications, and Adverse Pregnancy Outcomes: The Hordaland Homocysteine Study," *American Journal of Clinical Nutrition* 71(4) (2000): 962–8.
10. P. Ventura, et al., "Hyperhomocysteinemia and Related Factors in 600 Hospitalized Elderly Subjects," *Metabolism* 50(12) (2001): 1466–71.
11. K. Robinson et al., "Hyperhomocysteinemia and Low Pyridoxal Phosphate: Common and Independent Reversible Risk Factors for Coronary Artery Disease," *Circulation* 92(10) (1995): 2825–30.
12. F. Landgren et al., "Plasma Homocysteine in Acute Myocardial Infarction: Homocysteine-lowering Effect of Folic Acid," *Journal of Internal Medicine* 237 (1995): 381–8.
13. Harvard Medical School, "Harvard Men's Health Watch informs seniors about special nutrition needs," Harvard Health Publications, press release (May 26, 2004), www.health.harvard.edu/press_releases/mens_health_nutrition_information.htm.
14. M. den Heijer et al., "Hyperhomocysteinemia as a Risk Factor for Deep-vein Thrombosis," *New England Journal of Medicine* 334(12) (1996): 759–62.
15. P.M. Ridker et al., "Inflammation, Aspirin, and the Risk of Cardiovascular Disease in Apparently Healthy Men," *New England Journal of Medicine* 336(14) (1997): 973–9.

16. M. Di Napol, F. Papa, and V. Bocola, "C-reactive Protein in Ischemic Stroke: an Independent Prognostic Factor," *Stroke* 32(4) (2001): 917–24.
17. A.C. St. Pierre et al., "Effect of Plasma C-Reactive Protein Levels in Modulating Risk of Coronary Heart Disease Associated with Small, Dense, Low-Density Lipoproteins in Men (The Quebec Cardiovascular Study)," *American Journal of Cardiology* 91 (2003): 5–58.
18. K.M. Dalessandri, "Reduction of Lipoprotein(a) in Post-menopausal Women," *Archives of Housernl Medicine* 161(5) (2001): 772–3.
19. A.K. Bordia, "The Effect of Vitamin C on Blood Lipids, Fibrinolytic Activity and Platelet Adhesiveness in Patients with Coronary Artery Disease," *Atherosclerosis* 35(2) (1980): 1817.
20. K. Nyyssonen et al., "Vitamin C Deficiency and Risk of Myocardial Infarction: Prospective Population Study of Men from Eastern Finland," *British Medical Journal* 314(7081) (1997): 634–8.
21. S. Devaraj et al., "Alpha-tocopherol Supplementation Decrease Serum C-reactive Protein and Monocyte Interleukin-6 Levels in Normal Volunteer and Type-2 Diabetic Patients," *Free Radical Biology and Medicine* 29 (2000): 790–2.
22. J. Wang et al., "Multicenter Clinical Trial of the Serum Lipid-Lowering Effects of a Monascus Purpureus (Red Yeast) Rice Preparation From Traditional Chinese Medicine," *Current Therapeutic Research* 58(12) (1997): 964–78.
23. L. Patrick and M. Uzick, "Cardiovascular Disease: C-Reactive Protein and Inflammatory Disease Paradigm: HMG-COA Reductase Inhibitors, Alpha-tocopherol, Red Yeast Rice, and Olive Oil Polyphenols: A Review of the Literature," *Alternative Medical Review* 6 (2001): 248–71.
24. "Wobenzym as an Antiedematous Drug in Vascular Reconstructive Surgical Procedures: Efficacy and Tolerance," Mucos, web article, www.mucos.cz/eng/kardio/woabe.html.
25. V.N. Kovalenko, I.K. Sledzevskaya, E.N. Ryabokon, T.I. Gavrilenko, and A.I. Terzov, "New Approaches to Modern Cardiology Based on Systemic Enzyme Therapy," *International Journal of Immunotherapy* 17(2/3/4) (2001): 101–11.
26. C. Suarez et al., "The Prognostic Value of Analytical Hemorheological Factors in Stroke," *Review of Neurology* 24(126) (1996): 190–2.
27. T. Hiraga et al., "Hypertriglyceridemia, but not Hypercholesterolemia, is Associated with Alterations of Fibrinolytic System," *Hormone and Metabolic Research* 28(11) (1996): 603–6.
28. C.J. Packard et al., "Lipoprotein-associated Phospholipase A2 as an Independent Predictor of Coronary Heart Disease," *New England Journal of Medicine* 343(16) (2000): 1148–55.
29. A.K. Bordia, "The Effect of Vitamin C on Blood Lipids and Fibrinolytic Activity and Platelet Adhesiveness in Patients with Coronary Artery Disease," *Atherosclerosis* 35(2:180) (1980): 1–87.
30. S.K. Chutani and A. Bordia, "The Effect of Fried Versus Raw Garlic on Fibrinolytic Activity in Man," *Atherosclerosis* 38 (1981): 417–21.

31. R. Saynor and T. Gillott, "Changes in Blood Lipids and Fibrinogen with a Note on Safety in a Long Term Study on the Effects of n-3 Fatty Acids in Subjects Receiving Fish Oil Supplements and Followed for Seven Years," *Lipids* 27(7) (1992): 533–8.
32. P.C. Calder, "N-3 Polyunsaturated Fatty Acids and Inflammation: From Molecular Biology to the Clinic," *Lipids* 38(4:340) (2003): 3–52.
33. R.B. Arora et al., Anti-inflammatory Studies on *Curcuma Longa* (Turmeric). *Indian Journal of Medical Research* 59(8) (1971): 1289–95.
34. J.A. Duke, *The Green Pharmacy* (New York: St. Martin's, 1998).
35. A. Leitchle et al., "Alpha-tocopherol Distribution in Lipoproteins and Anti-inflammatory Effects Differ Between CHD Patients and Healthy Subjects," *Journal of the American College of Nutrition* 25(5) (2006):420–8.

12

Myths and Truths About Your Diet

The American Heart Association (AHA) recommends that individuals not consume more than 30% of their calories from fats, with only 10% (or less) coming from saturated fats. (Margarine is preferred over butter, and due to their high-fat content, nuts must then be limited to three or fewer servings a week.) They also recommend up to 11 servings of grains a day.

Myth: The AHA Diet is Good for You.

A recent systematic review of intervention trials based on the AHA diet showed only a slight benefit, which disappeared altogether when a trial that used fish was excluded.[1] This should come as no surprise since we've already established that low-fat diets don't alter mortality rates associated with CAD. In fact, it's been shown that low-fat, low-cholesterol diets cause a whole host of health problems, including increased death, depression, suicide, and hormonal imbalances. (Read more about this in chapter 7.)

Studies show that eating four or more servings of nuts a week lowers the risk of CAD by 50%![2] But the AHA is so fat phobic, they don't realize that restricting dietary nut intake actually contributes to CAD.

As for the margarine recommendation, a Harvard study found

that women who ate four or more teaspoons of margarine a day had a 50% greater risk of developing heart disease than did those who rarely ate margarine.[3] That's because margarine is loaded with trans fats, which poison the body, as I'll explain later in this chapter.

The diet advocated by the AHA also encourages the overconsumption of carbohydrates, especially whole grains. While I applaud the recommendation of eating whole grains (which are much more nutritious) instead of processed grains (which most Americans consume), the AHA neglects to tell you that increasing your grain intake may also increase the amount of inflammatory omega-6 arachidonic acids you store. It will surely increase the imbalance of omega-6 to omega-3 ratio for most Americans, who usually don't get enough omega-3 essential fatty acids in their diets.

It is ironic that the AHA recommends we reduce our fat intake in order to reduce the amount of triglycerides (blood fats) supposedly associated with an increased risk of heart disease. Because by increasing our carbohydrate intake, we actually increase, not reduce, our triglyceride levels. In fact, there is evidence that CAD is *encouraged* to progress in people on the high-carbohydrate AHA diet.[4]

Myth: It's Fat That Makes Us Fat.

Not hardly. It's all those carbs the AHA is throwing at us!

The Value of Carbs: Carbohydrates are essential for proper metabolic functions. They are quick sources of glucose, a sugar that generates energy for the body to run properly. Glucose is the brain's only food, and the brain refuses to go hungry without a fight. If you've ever experienced a hypoglycemic (low blood sugar) state, you know what I mean. Hypoglycemia can trigger fatigue, irritability, anger, anxiety, depression, and mental lethargy. You might crave sugar. Or the brain will pull the glucose out of muscle and fat tissue (this is what happens on low-carb diets, and why muscle mass is often lost on these diets).

Keeping the body fueled with adequate amounts of glucose is a challenge, since the liver, which stores "backup glucose" called glycogen, can only accommodate the equivalent of two cups of pasta. This must be replaced every five hours. The key is to not go too long without eating and to balance your intake of carbohydrates, fats, and proteins. Too many carbs (such as 11 servings a day) can be quite damaging.

The Challenge of Carbs: There is a growing body of research that indicates that excess carbohydrate—especially simple carbohydrate—intake increases triglyceride levels. Triglycerides are fatty acids that exist in food as well as in the body. Most fat in our bodies and in the food we eat is in the form of triglycerides: three fatty-acid chains attached to a glycerol molecule.

Calories ingested in a meal and not immediately used as fuel by the body are then converted to triglycerides and transported to fat cells to be stored for later use. Triglycerides are not derived from the fats we eat but from excess carbohydrate (especially sugar) intake! Having these excess triglycerides in plasma is called hypertriglyceridemia, and it has been associated with an increased risk of coronary artery disease in some people. (Elevated triglycerides may sometimes be a consequence of other diseases, such as uncontrolled diabetes.)

The new cholesterol guidelines recommend triglyceride levels be kept at or below 100. This is an absurd number, difficult to meet without a major change to current diet principles. Most Americans are destined to statin-drug therapy in an attempt to lower their apparently dangerous triglyceride levels. What a recipe for disaster!

The real culprit in increased triglyceride levels is the excess consumption of simple carbohydrates. These carbs are called simple because they have only one or two connected sugar molecules. Simple carbohydrates include fructose (found in fruits), galactose (in dairy products), maltose (starches/grains), levulose (table/cane sugar), glucose (grape and corn syrup), sucrose (table, cane, or beet sugar), and lactose (milk). (cow's milk is very high in sugar; please don't worry about the fat in milk).

Added sweeteners are the sneakiest culprits of the simple-carb epidemic. Half of all carbohydrates consumed in the United States are in the form of foods filled with added sweeteners. Because of this, the average American consumes over 125 pounds of sugar a year! And she doesn't even know she's eating it.

Why are simple carbs so damaging to our system? It's because of our body's reaction to them. When we eat a meal that contains large amounts of carbohydrates, especially simple carbohydrates, our blood-sugar levels begin to rise. The blood sugar is in the form of glucose, which is what all our food becomes in order to be used for energy. Unfortunately, we only need so much glucose, and too much at once causes it to build up in our blood. The body must counter this rapid rise in blood glucose by releasing the hormone insulin. Insulin then shunts excess carbohydrates into the cells, where it is stored as fat.

The role of insulin, produced by the pancreas, traces its roots back to a time when man's very survival depended on bodily reserves of fat, which was used by the body as fuel when wild game was in short supply. Centuries ago, before man was agriculturally inclined, our diet consisted of wild animals, berries, nuts, and fruits. These were not consumer-friendly times! Often, man himself was being hunted. He couldn't walk into the local grocery store and purchase that night's dinner. These hunters and gatherers would go days, sometimes weeks, without eating. During these lean times, glucose would be stored in fat tissue to serve as bodily fuel.

In today's fast food, "eat till you flop" world, insulin's efficiency leads to unwanted weight gain. Because of insulin's actions of helping turn glucose into fat, even fat-free foods, eaten to excess, turn into fat. And simple carbohydrates are the *worst* offenders. Not only do too many of them cause unwanted weight gain by turning into fat, they also contribute to arteriosclerosis, depression, and malnutrition.

Truth: You Body Can Only Take So Much Junk Food

If you need evidence for this truth, consider the epidemic of hyperinsulinemia in our country.

Insulin's primary function is to regulate blood sugar levels. It puts the sugar where it belongs (in the cells) and stimulates the liver to release glycogen (stored sugar) when levels are low. Excess blood sugar is transported out of the bloodstream and into the cells where it is stored as fat. The relationship between glucose, glucagon, and insulin is a self-regulating system that serves us well until our metabolism starts to slow down.

Years of eating excess carbohydrates—especially simple carbohydrates—and the effects of metabolic aging begin to take their toll in our mid-30s and 40s. By this time, too many of us have used up the storage space in the cells of our bodies. (Are you overweight? All that fat takes up a lot of cell space). Once full, these cells won't allow any more sugar in. The body attempts to remedy the sugar-storage problem by reducing the cells' insulin receptors. Unfortunately, this sends a message to the pancreas to release even more insulin. This results in hyperinsulinemia, and it is the beginning of type-2 diabetes. (Type-1 diabetes is a completely different disease where the body's insulin-producing cells in the pancreas have been destroyed for some reason.)

In this hyperinsulinemic condition, there is more insulin produced than is required by the amount of glucose present in the bloodstream. Why does the pancreas make so much insulin? One theory is that when high concentrations of sugar enter the blood stream so rapidly, the healthy pancreas overreacts.

For example, you eat a candy bar. The sugar in the candy bar enters the small intestine and is rapidly broken down; since there are not many nutrients to process and direct, the process goes like a flash. All that resulting glucose is then dumped into the bloodstream. The pancreas, in response to a large wave of glucose being released so fast, oversecretes insulin. The excess insulin consequently lowers the blood sugar within a short period of time to a hypoglycemic (low blood sugar) state. The individual then naturally craves more sugar, and the cycle is repeated.

Increased insulin levels, decreased insulin cell receptors, and cells stuffed full of fat prevent sugar from reaching its intended destination, the cells. Instead, the sugar remains in the bloodstream where it can cause damage to the arterial walls and lead to high blood pressure, arteriosclerosis, high blood-lipid levels, heart disease, and type-2 diabetes. Of course, some people have a genetic predisposition to type-2 diabetes and might not be able to avoid developing it to some extent. But many Americans with the dreaded disease could have avoided it if they had only known what their diet was doing to their bodies!

A Better Way: In contrast to simple carbohydrates, complex carbohydrates offer a wealth of nutritional value. Complex carbs are made up of long chains of three or more sugars. Examples of complex carbohydrates include most vegetables, unprocessed (whole) grains, and legumes.

Another way to judge your carbohydrate choices is through the use of the glycemic index (GI). The GI is a measurement of how much and how quickly a food elevates the circulating blood sugar of the normal person. Generally, the GI index follows the logic that the more complex a carbohydrate, the slower it is broken down. However, the body is a complicated system, and this is not always the case. The GI index has been developed by actually testing every food and recording how it is uniquely processed. The lower the GI, the slower the absorption, and the less stress put on your body. Some foods and their GI category are shown below as an example of how tricky those high-GI foods can be to spot. A high ("H") GI food has a rating of 70 or more. Moderate ("M") GI foods range from 56 to 69. A rating of 55 or below qualifies a food as low ("L") GI. A more complete list is available from many sources, including the easy-to-access www.lowglycemicdiet.com. For a more thorough discussion and complete resources on the topic, visit the official web site of the glycemic-index database: www.glycemicindex.com.

Breakfast Cereals
H: Cheerios
M: Raisin Bran
L: All Bran

Crackers
H: nearly all of them
M: some crispbreads
L: none I know of

Snacks
H: pretzels
M: corn chips
L: nuts

Fruits
H: watermelon
M: apricots
L: strawberries

Pasta
H: gnocchi
M: rice pasta
L: most others

Breads
H: whole-wheat bread
M: whole-wheat pita
L: stone-ground whole-wheat bread

Vegetables
H: pumpkin
M: corn
L: nearly all the rest

Rice
H: white rice
M: basmati rice
L: brown rice

Potatoes
H: baked potatoes
M: new potatoes
L: sweet potatoes

Avoid or severely reduce all high-GI foods and go easy on moderate-GI foods. Avoid the obvious culprits like white and red potatoes, white rice, most bread, anything made with corn (including popcorn), and anything with refined sugar (most baked goods). Avoid honey, maple syrup, corn syrup, sucrose (table sugar), and fructose (fruit juice). Even though some of these have a lower GI, they are still simple sugars and can rush your system with glucose. For sweetening, use plant-based sweeteners like stevia or fructoligosaccharide (FOS). Both are available at health food stores.

Diabetics might need to resort to artificial sweeteners; saccharine (Sweet-N-Low) and sucralose (Splenda) are preferable to aspartame (NutraSweet). To go completely no-carb, choose the tablet form of these sweeteners; the granular form does contain some carbs.[5]

Myth: Good Carbs are for Everyone all the Time

The fact is that many people are carbohydrate intolerant. Their cells have become full of stored carbohydrates (turned into fat) and can't effectively metabolize much more. Intolerance to carbohydrates may cause fatigue, mental lethargy, confusion, depression, headaches, bloating, indigestion, and weight gain. A two-week trial on a low-carbohydrate diet is an easy way to see if you are carb intolerant. (Individuals with low serotonin levels should be careful not to reduce their carbohydrate intake too quickly.)[6]

The Two-Week Low-Carb Challenge

For two weeks, eliminate all breads, pastas, cereals, milk, fruit juices, simple carbohydrate snacks, potatoes, cakes, cookies, and other sweets. Stick to low-glycemic foods, and try to keep total carbohydrate intake at or below 20 grams a day.

If after two weeks on this diet you feel better, then you are most likely carbohydrate intolerant, and this is the right diet for you. If after two weeks you are feeling good and have lost some weight, keep it up for another 2–4 weeks, and see how you feel.

Most individuals will do well on this test diet. Others with extremely low serotonin levels may bottom out and feel miserable. It's not uncommon for people to have sugar-withdrawal symptoms on this diet, but over time, the cravings will subside.

Long-term use of this diet can cause some unwanted side effects. As described above, when carb intake is low, protein stored in muscles may be needed to supply additional glucose for the brain. When the body starts to burn up stored proteins, it must conserve the essential proteins. It does this by producing a substitute fuel from the breakdown of fatty acids. This process yields a by-product known as ketones. The kidneys then attempt to flush out these ketones and, in so doing, also rid the body of excess water. That's why the initial rapid weight loss experienced on low-carb diets is due to water loss. Continuing a low-carbohydrate diet *will* start to burn up excess fat (and cause weight loss), but it also increases the risk of a ketonic state. In this state, the blood more acidic than it should be. This increased acidity can cause headaches, bad breath, dizziness, fatigue, and nausea.

The body simply shouldn't be subjected to long-term ketonic states; it's not healthy. It's best to try a two-week low-carb challenge test followed by a moderate (balanced) carbohydrate- management diet. I've found that a diet that avoids high glycemic foods and provides a balanced intake of 40% complex carbohydrates, 30% protein, and 30% fat is the healthiest way to lose weight. (These are rough percentages only, since I don't recommend counting calories or percentages but rather making wise choices on a day-to-day basis.)

What's the Best Diet for Me?

The healthiest diet is one based on whole, unprocessed foods. This means avoiding most prepackaged and all overly processed foods (including pretzels, sugar-loaded cereals, cookies, cakes, bagels, doughnuts, pastries, enriched breads, potato chips, corn chips, and margarine). Try to eat a diet full of raw or live foods, preferably organic. Include beef, chicken, and turkey (preferably grass-fed and hormone-free) as well as preservative- and additive-free eggs, cheese, and butter. Eat mercury-free, cold-water fish; raw nuts and seeds (such as almonds, walnuts, cashews, sunflower, pumpkin, and pecans); and a variety of fruits and vegetables. Shop the outside aisles of your grocery store first. That's where you'll find the fresh produce, refrigerated foods, dairy, and meats. Shoot for 2–3 servings of fruit, 3–4 servings of vegetables, and 2–3 servings of meat each day. Use natural, cold-expeller-pressed olive oil or canola oil for dressings and cooking.

Try not to be concerned with percentages or even calories. Simply reduce the processed foods you eat and increase the amount of whole foods you consume each day. You might be shocked at the results.

Myth: Vegetable Oils are Good for You

The AHA has promoted this, since *natural* vegetable oils are unsaturated (double-bonded). But these fats are poisoned by heating them up and hydrogenating them into trans fatty acids. Trans fatty acids prevent the omega-6 and omega-3 essential fatty acids from attaching to their receptors on cell membranes. This makes the membranes, which regulate what goes into and out of a cell, impermeable. Because nutrients can't get in and toxins can't get out, the membranes begin to die.

Processed vegetable oils, devoid of healthy essential fatty acids, are primarily toxic, trans fatty acids in a bottle.[7] These refined oils are devoid of lecithin, beta carotene, essential fatty acids, and the antioxidant vitamin E through the processes of deodorization, bleaching, and hydrogenation. Hydrogenation means adding hydrogen atoms to polyunsaturated oils for the purpose of creating solid saturated fats like margarine. To create these facts, natural oils are heated under pressure for 6–8 hours at 248–410 degrees F and reacted with hydrogen gas by using a metal like nickel or copper (both of which have been linked to mental depression and fatigue).

Truth: Trans Fats Should be Completely Avoided

Individuals increase their risk of developing coronary heart disease by a whopping 25% for every 2% increase in trans fatty acids.[8] And a 2% increase in trans fatty acid intake increases the risk of developing type-2 diabetes by 39%.[9]

Food labels must list trans fatty acids in the nutrition information. For healthy choices, look for labels that say "made from cold-expeller-pressed oils." Avoid margarine, enriched breads, foods cooked with vegetable oils (unless they state "expeller pressed" or have 0 trans fats listed), and hydrogenated or partially hydrogenated oils. Cook with olive oil or canola oil, both of which can withstand a higher cooking temperature before turning into trans fats. I recommend extra-virgin expeller-pressed olive oil.

Myth: Saturated Fact is Bad for You

It might come as a big surprise, but there is *no* evidence that saturated fats are bad for health, and there is plenty of evidence that saturated fats prevent both CVD and stroke.[10] In fact, the fatty acids found in clogged arteries are mostly *unsaturated* (74%), of which 41% are polyunsaturated.[11] Still, the AHA recommends reducing your intake of saturated fats and increasing your intake of unsaturated fats as insurance against heart disease. They aren't sadists; they're just behind the times.

In the early 1920s, coronary heart disease was rare in America. In fact, the inventor of the EKG was advised by his colleagues at Harvard University to avoid cardiology and concentrate on a more profitable branch of medicine.

Of course, we know that heart disease did not remain a novelty. By the mid-50s, it was the leading cause of death among Americans. What I find interesting is that if we go back and trace the increase in heart disease, we also see an increased use of polyunsaturated vegetable oils and the reduction of saturated fats. Over the past 60 years, Americans have steadily reduced their consumption of animal-based saturated fats. While consumption of cholesterol actually rose 1%, saturated fat consumption was reduced from 83% of total fats to 62% over this period. While saturated fats were decreased, polyunsaturated fats increased. This was especially true for trans fats, which increased during this period by over 400%. Our sugar consumption increased by 60%.[12,13]

We need to realize that saturated fats should be a healthy part of our diet! For one thing, they are necessary for proper absorption of calcium.[14] These valuable fats also help protect the liver from alcohol and other toxins.[15,16] They enhance the immune system.[17] And, saturated fats help with the retention and utilization of essential fatty acids.[18,19]

Saturated fats are the preferred foods for the heart, which is why the fat around the heart muscle is highly saturated[20,21] and why the excess intake of polyunsaturated fats has been linked to such health conditions as heart disease, cancer, obesity, depression, and immune deficiency disorder.

Various nutritional experts have voiced their opinions on the fact that saturated fats aren't harmful to our health.[22] Whole foods (including whole meats) have been sustaining humans for centuries. The less we rely on processed foods, the healthier we are. Avoiding animal fat is not only unreasonable; it's unhealthy. We need the fats that these animals provide.

The body needs a combination of saturated and polyunsaturated fats. But when polyunsaturated fats acids are subjected to modern processing methods, they tend to become oxidized or rancid.[23] These polyunsaturated fats create free radicals, the dangers of which are explained in chapter 11.

What about Vegetarians?

All my feelings about saturated fats aside, I know that there are many healthy vegetarians out there. I'm a recovering vegetarian myself. Yes, a vegetarian diet can be healthy. And yes, the current handling of livestock is inhumane. Still, a vegetarian diet is not right for the majority of people. It is usually loaded with processed carbohydrates and omega-6-rich foods. It is also very difficult to get enough protein and fat from a vegetarian diet. This is especially true for those vegetarians who don't eat any animal products, including dairy and fish. I'm not saying a vegetarian diet is necessarily unhealthy; it's just difficult.

If you're a vegetarian, reduce your simple sugars and consume more balanced proteins. Hopefully, you're getting enough fat in your diet and/or taking omega-3 fatty acids. By avoiding animal products, you are helping to reduce the amount of arachidonic acid in your body. However, if you don't consume enough omega-3 fatty acids, you'll have a imbalanced ratio that may increase your risk for certain health conditions we've already covered.

We've covered a lot of ground in this book so far. I hope that you're beginning to realize how important diet, antioxidants, and nutritional supplements are in preventing and restoring poor health. The best defense is an aggressive offense. In the next chapter, I'll be discussing another safe, effective, and proven therapy to reduce CAD.

Notes

1. L. Hooper et al., "Dietary Fat Intake and Prevention of Cardiovascular Disease," *British Medical Journal* 322(7289) (2001): 757–63.
2. G.E. Fraser et al., "A Possible Protective Effect of Nut Consumption on Risk of Coronary Heart Disease: The Adventist Health Study," *Archives of Internal Medicine* 152(7) (1992): 1416–24.
3. Harvard School of Public Health, "Fats and Cholesterol: Out With the Bad, In With the Good," *The Nutrition Source,* web article (2002), www.hsph.harvard.edu/nutritionsource/what-should-you-eat/fats-full-story/index.html.
4. M.A. Denke, "Metabolic Effects of High-protein, Low-carbohydrate Diets," *American Journal of Cardiology* 88(1) (2001): 59–61.
5. Even though "less than one" carb is listed per serving for granular artificial sweeteners, these small servings can add up, causing a rise in the blood sugar of type-1 diabetics, who can't even process small amounts of carbs without injected insulin.
6. This is because carbohydrates stimulate the release of insulin, and insulin allows the amino acid tryptophan to cross the blood-brain barrier where it then turns into serotonin.
7. R.P. Mensink et al., "Effect of Dietary Cis and Trans Fatty Acids on Serum Lipoprotein[a] Levels in Humans," *Journal of Lipid Research* 33: 1493–1501.
8. C.M. Oomen et al., "Association Between Trans Fatty Acid Intake and 10-year Risk of Coronary Heart Disease in the Zutphen Elderly Study: a Prospective Population-based Study," *Lancet* 357(9258) (2001): 746–51.
9. J. Salmeron et al., "Dietary Fat Intake and Risk of Type 2 Diabetes in Women," *American Journal of Clinical Nutrition* 73(6) (2001): 1019–26.
10. A. Ottoboni and F. Ottoboni, *The Modern Nutritional Diseases: And How to Prevent Them* (Amazon.com, 2002), 36–7.
11. C. Felton et al., "Dietary Polyunsaturated Fatty Acids and Composition of Human Aortic Plaques," *Lancet* 344 (1994): 1195.
12. D. Groom, "Population Studies of Atherosclerosis," *Annals of Internal Medicine* 55(1) (1961): 51–62
13. W.F. Enos et al., "Pathogenesis of Coronary Disease in American Soldiers Killed in Korea," *Journal of the American Medical Association* 158 (1955): 912.
14. B.A. Watkins and M.F. Seifert, "Food Lipids and Bone Health" in *Food Lipids and Health,* ed. R.E. McDonald and D.B. Min (New York: Marcel Dekker, 1996) 101.
15. A.A. Nanji et al., "Dietary Saturated Fatty Acids: A Novel Treatment for Alcoholic Liver Disease," *Gastroenterology* 109(2) (1995): 547–54.

16. Y.S. Cha and D.S. Sachan, "Opposite Effects of Dietary Saturated and Unsaturated Fatty Acids on Ethanol-pharmacokinetics, Triglycerides and Carnitines," *Journal of the American College of Nutrition* 13(4) (1994): 338–43.
17. J.J. Kabara, "The Pharmacological Effects of Lipids," paper presented at The American Oil Chemists Society, Champaign, Illinois (1978), 1–14.
18. M.L. Garg et al., *FASEB Journal* 2(4) (1988): A852.
19. R.M. Oliart Ros et al, "Meeting Abstracts," AOCS Proceedings, Chicago (May 1998): 7.
20. L.D. Lawson and F. Kummerow, "Beta-Oxidation of the Coenzyme A Esters of Vaccenic, Elaidic, and Petroselaidic Acids by Rat Heart Mitochondria," *Lipids* 14 (1979): 501–3.
21. M.L. Garg, "Means of Delivering Recommended Levels of Long Chain n-3 Polyunsaturated Fatty Acids in Human Diets," *Lipids* 24(4) (1989): 334–9.
22. Sally Fallon, *Nourishing Traditions: The Cookbook That Challenges Politically Correct Nutrition and The Diet Dictocrats* (Winona Lake, IN: NewTrends, 1999).
23. Edward R. Pinckney and Cathey Pinckney, *The Cholesterol Controversy* (Los Angeles: Sherbourne, 1973), 127–31.

13

Chelation Therapy and Heavy-Metal Toxicity

You might be able to discuss vitamin and mineral replacement therapy with your conventional cardiologist, but mention chelation ("key-lay-shun") therapy, and you're sure to get an earful of venomous prattle about how it doesn't work and how dangerous it is. This is in spite of the fact that not one single person in 40 years has died using this therapy, and tens of thousands of patients die from unnecessary bypass surgery every year.

One conventional medical author put it this way (my paraphrase): Doctors who promote chelation are nothing but snake-oil salesmen. Recent studies have shown that chelation therapy doesn't reduce plaque, improve blood flow, or remove much of anything from the arteriosclerotic artery. And the therapy isn't without risk. It is dangerous and expensive, costing up to $3,000 for a series of I.V. sessions.

I find these comments interesting, since bypass surgery costs well over $50,000, hasn't been shown to increase lifespan in 95% of those who have the procedure, and carries several risks—including an up to 10% death rate. In contrast, chelation has been proven to increase blood flow and reduce the risk of mortality, not for cardiac disorders only but for many illnesses, including cancer.

Intravenous (I.V.) chelation therapy was first introduced in

1948 as a treatment for lead (a heavy metal) poisoning. Happily, physicians administering EDTA for lead poisoning found that their patients with CAD experienced a dramatic reduction in their symptoms! This included a reduction in chest pain and increased exercise tolerance.[1]

Most conventional doctors erroneously believe that EDTA chelation therapy has no documented scientific proof, but this could be no further from the truth. In fact there are over 1,800 scientific journal articles published on chelation therapy. In the past 40 years, over 1 million patients have been chelated with EDTA therapy.[2]

Dr. Elmer Cranton writes about his study that followed post-chelation patients over 18 years and showed that their mortality from cancer decreased by 90%.[3] The study was reviewed by the University of Zurich, which didn't find a single flaw.

EDTA, the chemical used for chelation therapy, is safe. In fact, it is much safer than aspirin![4] According to Dr. Elmer Cranton, author of *Bypassing Bypass Surgery*[5] and *A Textbook on EDTA Chelation Therapy,*[6] every chelation study has been favorable, even the one the conventional doctor above mentioned. What's more, Dr. Cranton, a graduate of Harvard Medical School, writes that 90% of his patients have improved after receiving chelation therapy. He'd have to be one heck of a "snake-oil salesman" to pull that off!

A 1993 meta-analysis looked at all the studies on chelation therapy up until that time. The analysis showed that 87% of the 22,765 patients in the studies showed a favorable response to chelation therapy.[7] That is pretty impressive, considering that many of these folks are the sickest of the sick. They have had numerous surgeries and/or have been told that traditional medicine has nothing left to offer them.

I remember many of these same patients who presented to my clinic for chelation therapy. They had been told to put their affairs in order; they didn't have very long to live. They had been to numerous other doctors, had previous life-threatening surgeries, and often had been on toxic medications for a number of years. They got better—some even well—after receiving chelation therapy. So obviously, I'm a fan of chelation therapy. I've had over 40 chelation treatments myself and know firsthand how helpful it can be in restoring a person's vitality. I've seen *miracles* occur in many of the patients who had the therapy administered at my clinic.

What Is Chelation Therapy?

Chelation therapy uses a man-made amino acid known as ethylene diamine tetraacetic acid (EDTA) to bind to—or chelate (from the Greek for "claw")—potentially toxic heavy metals. Heavy metals create free radicals, contribute to lipid peroxidation (oxidation of LDL), and cause arterial damage. EDTA has been shown to reduce free-radicals in the blood.[8] That's because metallic ions are needed as catalysts for free radicals to proliferate in cellular tissues. These metallic ions can't carry out their destructive free-radical mechanisms in the presence of EDTA.[10] It's your body's truant officer, rounding up the troublemakers (heavy-metal hoodlums) and taking them away.

Chelation therapy has been clinically shown to have numerous positive health benefits:

- helps maintain reduced blood aggregation or clotting[10]
- improves peripheral circulation (in 100% of the 2,870 patients, in one study)[11]
- increases blood flow to the brain[12]
- improves mental function in patients with prior memory problems[13]
- improves capillary flow[14]
- decreases blood pressure[15]
- removes toxic heavy metals including lead, aluminum, cadmium, and others, which accumulate with age and are the catalyst for free radicals[16]
- decreases free-radical damage[17]
- protects the integrity of blood platelets, preventing clotting[18]

There are two main types of chelation therapy: I.V. and oral. The I.V.-chelation therapy, I'll admit, isn't the most pleasant activity you could engage in. It involves making yourself as comfortable as possible while hooked up to an I.V. and letting the EDTA do the work. I always tried to keep my patients entertained with reading materials, but no one likes to sit around with an I.V. in their arm. However, there is just no substitute for allowing the blood to be directly accessed with healing elements.

I.V.-chelation therapy is also quite costly. It's about $3,000 for 30 (typically three-hour) sessions. Of course, compared to drug therapy, which may run hundreds of dollars a month, or bypass surgery, which costs $50,000, I.V. chelation is a bargain. And it has proven itself to be a safe and effective way to prevent and reverse the ravages of CAD. However, for individuals who don't have the time or money to invest in I.V. EDTA therapy, oral chelation is a valid option. There have been numerous studies that validate the use of oral chelation therapy. And although there is still quite a bit of debate among oral- and I.V.-chelation doctors, oral chelation is gaining favor among many who, until recently, doubted its validity.

Unfortunately, oral EDTA is not as strong as I.V. chelation therapy. While 100% of I.V. EDTA is absorbed, only 18% of oral EDTA is absorbed.[19] Still, oral chelation is a good fit for those who want to prevent heart disease. I.V. chelation is better suited for those individuals with severe heart disease. Garry Gordan, M.D., is perhaps the best known spokesman for oral chelation therapy. He reports that oral chelation therapy is similar to I.V. therapy in that it too eliminates heavy metals, reduces lipid peroxides and free radicals, lowers cholesterol, lowers blood pressure, and helps prevent blood clots.[20] Although I've been slow to acknowledge the benefits of oral EDTA chelation, I'm fast becoming a strong supporter of this safe, frugal, and effective therapy.

The table below offers an overview of the two therapies.

THERAPY:	**Oral Chelation**	**I.V. Chelation**
ADMINISTRATION:	7.5 g. EDTA daily	1–3 sessions weekly
AMOUNT ADSORBED:	5–9 g. a week	3–9 g. a week
APPROXIMATE COST:	$65/month	$400–$1,200/month
BEST FOR:	prevention of CAD	treatment of CAD

Is EDTA safe? Well, it is used in a number of foods as a preservative (therefore, it is generally recognized as safe), and we are exposed to a rather large amount (15–50 mg.) of it every day. Given the fact that we are all exposed to and probably loaded with toxic heavy metals, we could help ourselves dearly by starting a heavy-metal detoxification program built around oral chelation.

What is Heavy-Metal Toxicity?

Heavy-metal toxicity is quite common in today's environment. Many of our everyday activities and products contribute to our toxic-level exposure to heavy metals. Many of these metals have been implicated in causing or contributing to such conditions as CAD, Alzheimer's, attention deficit disorder, depression, headache, hypertension, kidney failure, loss of hearing, fibromyalgia, chronic fatigue syndrome, and tingling in the extremities. Let's look at some of these metals and what they are doing to our bodies.

Aluminum toxicity has been linked to pre-senile dementia, Alzheimer's,[21,22] and fibromyalgia. Aluminum is found in some most deodorants, antacids, some flours, baking-soda toothpaste, processed cheeses, toothpastes, shampoos and conditioners, prescription and nonprescription drugs (such as buffered aspirin), aluminum drink cans, and aluminum cookware. I highly recommend you use only stainless steel cookware and avoid aluminum-lined (and lead-lined) cans. Switch to natural toothpaste, hair products, and deodorants; visit your local health-food store for a wide selection. *Never* take antacids that contain aluminum! Not only do they contain toxic aluminum, they block hydrochloric acid, which prevents the body from synthesizing essential nutrients like Vitamin B12 (a deficiency of Vitamin B12 can cause dementia, Alzheimer's, depression and fatigue). Antacids also don't allow you to absorb calcium. So if you are taking Tums as a source of calcium, you have been duped once again by big-brother drug.

Arsenic toxicity can cause central depression, headache, high fevers, decreased red blood cells, fatigue, diarrhea, and even death. Municipal or well water may get contaminated with arsenic. Arsenic toxicity has been correlated with tainted water supplies.[23]

Cadmium at elevated levels is associated with hypertension, kidney failure, loss of coordination, numbness or tingling in the hands or feet, and loss of hearing.[24] Common environmental sources for exposure include tobacco smoke and oil-based paints. A zinc deficiency exacerbates the toxic effects of cadmium toxicity.

Lead, in toxic doses, has numerous documented effects, including neurological disorders in children, chronic anemia, learning disturbances, and fatigue.[25] Common sources of lead in the environment are lead-based paints, drinking water, industrial contaminants, airborne emissions, and occupations involving metal work and printing. Lead absorption is higher when calcium intake is deficient.

Mercury toxicity can cause a wide variety of health problems, including chronic fatigue, stunted growth, mental depression, muscle and joint pain, and possibly brain damage. (Mercury can suppress selenium absorption, and selenium can block mercury absorption, as they compete to bind with sulfur enzyme centers.) Mercury toxicity shows up as a multitude of symptoms. Confusion and dementia, numbness in the extremities, fibromyalgia, allergies, and chronic infections are some of them. Mercury may also modify normal bacteria so that they become pathogenic (disease causing). It blocks the function of the nerve cells in the brain and peripheral nervous system, and it can trigger autoimmune responses. Detoxifying from mercury requires oral herbs, mineral supplements, and prescription oral or intravenous medications.

Mercury can come from farmed foods. That's because tons of toxic industrial wastes, including heavy metals, are being mixed with liquid agricultural fertilizers and dispersed across America's farmlands. Mercury enters the water as a natural process of off-gassing from the earth's crust. But it also comes from industrial pollution: the use of fossil fuels, fungicides, and some paints, and the production of chlorine, paper, and pulp. Since it's in the water, it is routinely found in large predatory fish such as swordfish, shark, salmon, and tuna.

However, the primary sources of chronic, low-level mercury exposure are dental amalgams (the silver-colored fillings). Amalgams contain a highly absorbable form of mercury that is very reactive and vaporizes at room temperature. Mercury would be poorly absorbed if taken orally, but the vapors are readily absorbed through the lungs and quickly pass the blood-brain barrier. Once inside a cell, unfortunately mercury is usually there to stay. It continually accumulates in the kidneys, neurological tissue (including the brain), and the liver. High levels of mercury exposure have also been found in the heart, thyroid, and pituitary tissues of dentists. Animal research has shown that within 24 hours of having a mercury/silver filling placed, mercury can be detected in the spinal fluid of the animal, and within 48 hours, it is implanted in the brain.

In patients who have symptoms of mercury toxicity, mercury amalgams should be removed by a dentist who has expertise in the particular problems of mercury poisoning. Some patients have had worsening of their symptoms when their fillings were removed without the care necessary to prevent increased mercury exposure.[26,27]

Nickel is not as toxic as many of the other metals. Nevertheless, it's associated with headaches, diarrhea, blue gums and lips, lethargy, insomnia, rapid heart rate, and shortness of breath.

Copper at elevated levels has been implicated in learning and mental disorders and may contribute to increased systolic blood pressure.[28,29]

How Do I Know If I'm Toxic?

Hair analysis offers a reliable, low-cost way of measuring heavy-metal exposure. Since hair filaments may be active for months, even years, hair analysis can even provide a history of exposure.[30] Hair analysis testing kits can be ordered through my office. (See the appendix for ordering information.)

Heavy metals are clearly dangerous to your health. Consider having a hair analysis and starting a detoxification program with oral or intravenous chelation therapy. For more information on chelation therapy, see the appendix.

Notes

1. M. Walker and G. Gordon, *The Chelation Answer* (Atlanta: Second Opinion, 1994), 4.
2. ibid.
3. Elmer Cranton, *Bypassing Bypass Surgery* (Charlottesville: Hampton Roads, 2001).
4. H. Foreman, "Toxics Side Effects of EDTA," *Journal of Chronic Disease* 16 (1963): 319–323.
5. (Charlottesville: Hampton Roads, 2001).
6. ibid.
7. Elmer Cranton, *Bypassing Bypass Surgery* (Charlottesville: Hampton Roads, 2001), 123.

8. D.W. Morel, J.R. Hessler, G.M. Chisolm, "Low-density Lipoprotein Cytotoxicity Induced Free Radical Peroxidation of Lipid," *Journal of Lipid Research* 24 (1983): 1070–6.
9. J. March, *Advanced Organic Chemistry Reactions, Mechanics, and Structure,* 2nd ed. (New York: McGraw-Hill, 1978): 620.
10. M. Walker and G. Gordon, *The Chelation Answer* (Atlanta: Second Opinion, 1994), 4.
11. ibid.
12. ibid.
13. ibid.
14. ibid.
15. ibid.
16. Elmer Cranton, *Bypassing Bypass Surgery* (Charlottesville: Hampton Roads, 2001).
17. ibid.
18. ibid.
19. B. Halstead and T. Rozema, *The Scientific Basis of EDTA Chelation Therapy*, 2nd ed. (Landrum: TRC, 1997).
20. M. Walker and G. Gordon, *The Chelation Answer* (Atlanta: Second Opinion, 1994), 4.
21. O. Knoll et al., "Consequences from EEG Findings and Aluminum Encephalopathy," *Trace Elements in Medicine* 8-s (1991): 18-s.
22. S. L. Rifat, "Aluminum Hypothesis Lives," *Lancet* 343 (1994): 3–4.
23. J. Goldsmith et al., "Evaluation of Health Implications of Elevated Arsenic in Well Water," *Water Research* 6 (1972): 1133-6.
24. L. Friberg et al., *Cadmium in the Environment,* 2nd ed. (Cleveland: CRC, 1974).
25. J.D. Sargent, A. Meveres, and M. Weitzman, "Environmental Exposure to Lead and Cognitive Deficits in Children," letter, *New England Journal of Medicine* 320(9) (1989): 595.
26. F.L. Lorscheider, M.J. Vimy, and A.O. Summers, "Mercury Exposure From "Silver" Tooth Fillings: Emerging Evidence Questions a Traditional Paradigm," *FASEB Journal* 9 (1995): 504–8.
27. M. Nylander, L. Frieberg, and B. Lind, "Mercury Concentrations in the Brain and Kidneys in Relation to Exposure from Dental Amalgam Fillings," *Swedish Dental Journal* 11 (1987): 179–187.
28. B. Rimland and G.E. Larson, "The Feingold Diet: An Assessment of the Reviews by Mattes, by Kavale and Forness and Others," *Journal of Learning Disabilities* 16 (1983): 1–7.
29. K. Lerch, "Copper Monoxygenases: Tyrosinase and Dopamine B-Monooxygenase," in *Metal Ions in Biological Systems* 13, H. Sigel, ed. (New York: Marcel Dekker, 1981).
30. T. Suzuki and R. Yamamoto, "Organic Mercury Levels in Human Hair With and Without Storage for Eleven Years," *Bulletin of Environmental Contamination and Toxicology* 28 (1928):186–8.

14

Putting It All Together

In this book, I have exposed the medical myths associated with cholesterol and heart disease. I've poked holes in the "all fat is bad for you" mantra. Hopefully, I've cured you of the fat phobia that has plagued the citizens of America for the past four decades.

Remember that cholesterol plays a valuable role in promoting optimal health. It is responsible for steroid hormones, helps regulate the cellular membranes, and is a potent antioxidant that helps protect us from free-radical damage. Free radicals are at the heart (no pun intended) of CAD.

Cholesterol neurosis has been advocated by our medical organizations, even though studies don't show that reducing cholesterol actually saves lives. Instead, this obsession with low cholesterol has led to an ever-increasing use of statin medications, which cause CoQ10 deficiencies. CoQ10 is needed by every cell in the body and especially by the heart cells.

The rise in statin medications has paralleled the rise in congestive heart failure. A coincidence? Many experts don't think so. And while the medical profession obsesses over the lack of studies to support alternative methods, only 20% of all medical therapies have been proven. Bypass surgery is not one of them. There has never been a double-blind study on bypass surgery, yet half a million Americans will undergo this risky procedure this year. Medical journals report that the majority of bypass and angioplasty surgery isn't warranted.

Conventional doctors still ridicule EDTA chelation therapy for being dangerous and ineffective. This is in spite of the fact that studies have proven it does extend life. Give me a break. This would be comical if it weren't for the fact that the fourth leading cause of death in the United States is from the side effects associated with drugs and surgical procedures, which these same doctors advocate. I don't make this stuff up. It's all in the medical journals.

What can you do to reduce your risk of CAD? First of all, quit being so stressed out about fats and cholesterol. Stress over your cholesterol numbers will kill you faster than the numbers will. Eat eggs, meat, and all the butter you want. Avoid hydrogenated oils and trans fatty acids. Make the few grains you eat whole grains. Eat as many whole foods as possible. Eat plenty of fruits and vegetables.

If you aren't convinced you need to take fish oil after reading this book, then I don't know what else I can say. I recommend everyone—yes, everyone—take a minimum of 2 g. of fish oil each day. Those with high blood pressure or advanced CAD may need to take up to 9 g. a day. By reducing your intake of vegetable oils (omega-6) and supplementing with fish oil (omega-3), you can reduce the inflammatory chemicals that inhabit your body.

Everyone should be taking a good optimal-daily-allowance multivitamin, which contain 200 to 300 times the recommended daily allowance (RDA). (This excludes "supplements" like One a Day and Centrum Silver.) The RDA—or, as I like to call it, recommended disease allowance—is just enough to keep you from getting scurvy. It won't be enough to squelch the millions of free radicals that invade your body each day.

If you have CAD or high blood pressure, take a minimum of 100 mg. of CoQ10 daily. Try to eat several servings of fruits and vegetables each day. Get a pill book at your local bookstore, and look up and read about all the medications you're taking. Look at the potential side effects. Even a 1% risk is important, since you might be one of the unlucky one percent. But don't stop taking your medications without discussing it with your doctor, and always wean off medications slowly.

Begin an exercise program. Start slowly by walking 15 minutes a day. Try to build up to one hour a day. Oh, you don't have time to exercise? You must make time. It's that important. It is certainly more important than watching TV or reading the paper, both of which have so much bad news that you can't help but feel stressed out, anyway.

In addition to changing your diet, taking fish oil, exercising, and taking a good optimal-daily-allowance multivitamin and mineral formula, consider the novel nutritional therapies mentioned in this book, including Cardio-Stolix (BP Support), nattokinase, wobenzyme, and others.

If you have CAD, have high blood pressure, or have had heart surgery (or just want to feel better), then consider doing a course of chelation therapy.

Well, you've done it. You've finished the book. Now I recommend you check out the appendix, which immediately follows this chapter. You'll also find information on vitamin supplements, oral- and I.V.-chelation resources, and other topics of interest.

All the best in your endeavors to be healthier and live longer.

Appendix

About Dr. Murphree

Dr. Murphree is the past founder and clinical director of a large, integrated medical practice located on the campus of Brookwood Hospital in Birmingham, Alabama. The practice was staffed with medical doctors, acupuncturists, nutritionists, herbalists, and chiropractors, and it specialized in combining traditional and alternative medicine to treat a variety of health conditions, including heart disease, diabetes, hypertension, fibromyalgia, and chronic fatigue syndrome.

Dr. Murphree speaks about heart disease, hypertension, fibromyalgia, chronic fatigue syndrome, and integrative medicine to doctors and the public throughout North America. He is the author of four other books: *Treating and Beating Fibromyalgia and Chronic Fatigue Syndrome, The Patient Self-Help Manual for Treating Fibromyalgia and Chronic Fatigue Syndrome, Treating and Beating Fibromyalgia and Chronic Fatigue Syndrome: A Manual for Non-Allopathic Doctors,* and *Treating and Beating Anxiety and Depression with Orthomolecular Medicine.*

Dr. Murphree received his undergraduate degree from The University of Alabama, Birmingham (1985). He received his doctor of chiropractic degree from Life College in Atlanta in 1990. He is a board-certified chiropractic physician and certified nutritional specialist (American Board of Certified Nutritional Specialist, 2000). In 2001, he sold his interest in the medical practice and opened his own nutrition-based clinical practice in Homewood, Alabama, where he currently sees patients.

Dr. Murphree can be contacted by calling 205-879-2383 or 1-888-884-9577 or through www.TreatingandBeating.com. His mailing address is 2700 Rogers Drive, Suite 204, Homewood, Alabama, 35209.

To receive Dr. Murphree's free monthly email newsletter, please register at www.TreatingandBeating.com. There, you can also find more information on heart disease and many other health issues.

Ordering Information

Dr. Murphree

- www.treatingandbeating.com
- 205-879-2383 or toll free 1-888-884-9577
- Contact Dr. Murphree for a free catalog or to place an order for many of the supplements mentioned in this book—including oral chelation supplements, optimal daily allowance multivitamin and mineral formulas, mercury-free fish oil, and other specially designed nutritional supplements.

Douglas Laboratories

- 1-800-245-4440
- Douglas Labs offers many of the products recommended in this book; they are available through your doctor's order.

Referrals to Doctors

For referrals to doctors of natural medicine, including a list of doctors using chelation therapy, contact the **American College for Advancement in Medicine** (714-583-7666 or www.ACAM.org) or the **American Association of Naturopathic Physicians** (206-323-7610 or www.naturopathic.org).

More information about recommended lab tests can be found at www.TreatingAndBeating.com.

Laboratories

Metametrix Clinical Laboratory

- www.metametrix.com
- 1-800-221-4640

Genova Diagnostics

- www.gsdl.com
- 1-800-522-4762

Additional Research on Cholesterol

At least eight different trials have used diet alone to treat coronary heart disease. The number of fatal and nonfatal heart attacks weren't significantly reduced in any of the following trials.

- Research Committee, "Low-fat Diet in Myocardial Infarction: A Controlled Trial," *Lancet* 2 (1965): 501–4.
- G.A. Rose, W.B. Thomson, and R.T. Williams, "Corn Oil in Treatment of Ischaemic Heart Disease," *British Medical Journal* i (1965): 1531–3.
- Research Committee to the Medical Research Council, "Controlled Trial of Soya-bean Oil in Myocardial Infarction," *Lancet* ii (1968): 693–700.
- S. Dayton et al., "A Controlled Clinical Trial of a Diet High in Unsaturated Fat in Preventing Complications of Atherosclerosis," *Circulation* 40(s2) (1969): 1–63.
- P. Leren, The Effect of Plasma Cholesterol Lowering Diet in Male Survivors of Myocardial Infarction: A Controlled Clinical Trial," *Acta Medica Scandinavica* s466 (1966): 1–92.
- J.M. Woodhill et al., "Low-fat, Low Cholesterol Diet in Secondary Prevention of Coronary Heart Disease," *Advances in Experimental Medicine and Biology* 109 (1978): 317–30.
- M.L. Burr et al., "Effects of Changes in Fat, Fish, and Fibre Intakes on Death and Myocardial Reinfarction: Diet and Reinfarction Trial (DART)," *Lancet* 2 (1989): 757–61.
- I.D. Frantz et al., "Test of Effect of Lipid Lowering by Diet on Cardiovascular Risk: The Minnesota Coronary Survey," *Arteriosclerosis* 9 (1989): 129–35.

The article below reported on the doctors' review of 16 trials using low cholesterol diet as a means to lower blood cholesterol levels. They concluded that the "step-1" (low-saturated-fat, low-cholesterol) diet lowered blood cholesterol by only 0%–4%.

- L.E. Ramsay, W.W. Yeo, and P.R. Jackson, "Dietary Reduction of Serum Cholesterol Concentration: Time to Think Again," *British Medical Journal* 303 (1991): 953–7.

Studies of African tribes have shown that intakes of enormous amounts of animal fat don't raise blood cholesterol levels. Many of these people have some of the lowest cholesterol levels ever recorded, despite diets high in animal products. The Samburu tribe eats about a pound of meat and drinks almost two gallons of raw milk each day. They consume more than twice the amount of animal fat than the average American, and yet their cholesterol is much lower, about 170 mg./dl.

- A.G. Shaper, "Cardiovascular Studies in the Samburu Tribe of Northern Kenya," *American Heart Journal* 63 (1962): 437–42.

Shepherds in Somalia consume almost a gallon and a half of camel milk each day, which amounts to almost one pound of butter fat. But their mean cholesterol is only about 150 mg./dl, far lower than that of most Western people.

- G.V. Mann, R.D. Shaffer, and H.H. Sandstead, "Cardiovascular Disease in the Masai," *Journal of Atherosclerosis Research* 4 (1964): 289–312.

Similar studies have been performed in other countries—including India, Poland, Guatemala, and the United States—all with the same result: no correlation between the level of cholesterol in the blood stream and the amount of atherosclerosis in the vessels.

- K.S. Mathur et al., "Serum Cholesterol and Atherosclerosis in Man," *Circulation* 23 (1961): 847–52.
- Z. Marek, K. Jaegermann, and T. Ciba, "Atherosclerosis and Levels of Serum Cholesterol in Postmortem Investigations," *American Heart Journal* 63 (1962): 768–74.
- J. MŽndez and C. Tejada, "Relationship Between Serum Lipids and Aortic Atherosclerotic Lesions in Sudden Accidental Deaths in Guatemala City," *American Journal of Clinical Nutrition* 20 (1967): 1113–7.
- H.S. Cabin and W.C. Roberts, "Relation of Serum Total Cholesterol and Triglyceride Levels to the Amount and Extent of Coronary Arterial Narrowing by Atherosclerotic Plaque in

Coronary Heart Disease," *American Journal of Medicine* 73 (1982): 227–34.

Researchers in Copenhagen found that among over 20,000 patients, only those with cholesterol levels in the top 5% were at risk of developing heart disease.

- E. Lindenstrom, G. Boysen, and J. Nyboe, "Influence of Total Cholesterol, High Density Lipoprotein Cholesterol, and Triglycerides on Risk of Cerbrovascular Disease: the Copenhagen City Heart Study," *British Medical Journal* 309 (1994): 11–15.

Several studies have found that low cholesterol may be worse than high cholesterol. When 19 studies—involving over 68,000 deaths—were reviewed by Professor David R. Jacobs and his coworkers from the Division of Epidemiology at the University of Minnesota, low cholesterol predicted an increased risk of dying from gastrointestinal and respiratory diseases.

- D. Jacobs et al., "Report of the Conference on Low Blood Cholesterol: Mortality Associations," *Circulation* 86, (1992): 1046–60.

Other researchers have made similar observations. One of the largest studies was conducted at UCLA Department of Medicine and Cardiomyopathy Center in Los Angeles. The study involved more than a thousand patients with severe congestive heart failure. After five years, 62% of the patients with cholesterol below 129 mg./l had died, but only half as many of the patients with cholesterol above 223 mg./l.

- T.B. Horwich et al., "Low Serum Total Cholesterol is Associated with Marked Increase in Mortality in Advanced Heart Failure," *Journal of Cardiac Failure* 8 (2002): 216–24.

Additional Research on Statin Drugs

The following study showed that prevastatin is only slightly better than placebo (sugar pill) in preventing a second heart attack.

- F.M Sacks et al., "The Effect of Pravastatin on Coronary Events After Myocardial Infarction in Patients with Average

Cholesterol Levels," *New England Journal of Medicine* 335 (1996): 1001–9.

An analysis of all the major controlled trials before the year 2000 found that long-term use of statins for primary prevention of heart disease produced a 1% greater risk of death over 10 years compared to a placebo.

- P.R. Jackson, "Statins for Primary Prevention: At What Coronary Risk is Safety Assured?" *British Journal of Clinical Pharmacology* 52 (2001): 439–46.

The Antihypertensive and Lipid-Lowering Treatment to Prevent Heart Attack Trial (ALLHAT) was the largest North American cholesterol-lowering trial ever and the largest trial in the world using Lipitor. Researchers followed 10,000 participants over a period of four years. They compared the use of Lipitor to "usual care" (maintaining proper body weight, not smoking, regular exercise, etc). Of the 5,170 subjects in the group that received Lipitor, 28% lowered their LDL cholesterol significantly. And of the 5,185 usual-care subjects (who didn't take Lipitor but focused on lifestyle), about 11% had a similar drop in LDL. Heart attack, heart disease, and death rates of the treatment group and controls after three or six years were nearly *identical.*

- The ALLHAT Officers and Coordinators for the ALLHAT Collaborative Research Group, "The Antihypertensive and Lipid-Lowering Treatment to Prevent Heart Attack Trial," *Journal of the American Medical Association* 288 (2002): 2998–3007.

The Heart Protection Study, carried out in 2002 at Oxford University (see 1, below), received widespread press coverage; researchers claimed "massive benefits" from cholesterol-lowering statin drugs, leading one commentator to call them "the new aspirin" (2, below). But as Dr. Ravnskov points out (3), the benefits were far from massive. Those who took simvastatin had an 87.1% survival rate after five years compared to an 85.4% survival rate for the controls, and these results were *independent* of the amount of cholesterol lowering (4).

1. Heart Protection Study Collaborative Group, "Heart Protection Study of Cholesterol Lowering With Simvastatin in 20,536 High-risk Individuals: a Randomised Placebo-controlled Trial." *Lancet* 360 (2002): 7–22.
2. Medical Research Council/British Heart Foundation's Heart Protection Study, "Life-saver: World's Largest Cholesterol-lowering Trial Reveals Massive Benefits for High-risk Patients." See a discussion by the American College of Cardiology at www.cardiosource.com/clinicaltrials/trial.asp?TrialID=468.
3. A. Kmietowicz, "Statins Are the New Aspirin, Oxford Researchers Say," *British Medical Journal* 323 (2001): 1145.
4. U. Ravnskov and C. Anton, "Statins as the New Aspirin," letter, *British Medical Journal* 324 (2002): 789. See a discussion at www.bmj.com/cgi/eletters/324/7340/789.

The Japanese Lipid Intervention Trial (J-LIT) of 2002 was a six-year study of 47,294 patients treated with the same dose of simvastatin. Patients were grouped by the amount of cholesterol lowering achieved. Some patients had no reduction in LDL levels; some had a moderate drop; and some had very large LDL reductions. The results show *no correlation* between the amount of LDL lowering and death rate at five years. Those with LDL cholesterol lower than 80 had the nearly *identical* death rate as those whose LDL was over 200.

• M. Matsuzaki et al., "Large Scale Cohort Study of the Relationship Between Serum Cholesterol Concentration and Coronary Events with Low-dose Simvastatin Therapy in Japanese Patients with Hypercholesterolemia," *Circulation Journal* 66(12) (2002): 1087–95.

In a meta-analysis of 44 trials involving almost 10,000 patients, the death rate was *identical* in each of the three groups: those taking atorvastatin (Lipitor), those taking other statins, and those taking no drugs at all for heart disease.

• H.S. Hecht and S.M. Harmon, "Statins in Prevention: Many Risks, Few Beneficiados!," *American Journal of Cardiology* 92 (2003): 670–6.

The Pravastatin or AtorVastatin Evaluation and Infection Study (PROVE-IT) was led by researchers at Harvard University Medical School and compared two statin drugs: Lipitor and Pravachol.

The study looked at 4,162 patients who had been in the hospital following a heart attack or unstable angina. Half were given Pravachol; half got Lipitor. Those taking Lipitor had a 32% greater reduction in LDL levels and a 16% reduction in all-cause mortality. The "striking benefit" was a 22% rate of death or further adverse coronary events in the Lipitor patients, compared to 26% in the Pravachol patients.

These are impressive numbers, but what did the study prove? Not that lowering LDL reduces mortality but that Lipitor is more effective at reducing LDL *and* at reducing mortality rates than is Pravachol. Neither drug, however, has been proven better than the therapies described in this book (but they are certainly more dangerous).

- C.P. Cannon et al., "Intensive versus Moderate Lipid Lowering with Statins after Acute Coronary Syndromes," *New England Journal of Medicine* 350(15) (2004): 1495–504.

More About Vitamin and Mineral Supplements

If you compare Centrum or One A Day vitamins to my Essential Therapeutics multivitamin and mineral formulas, you'll notice our specially designed vitamins have 50 times or even 100 times the recommended daily allowance (RDA). This is because the RDA is an outdated system that does not take into account the depletion of our nutrient-rich top soil, environmental pollutants, chemical food processing, the addition of artificial ingredients, and the increased demands placed on an individual's homeostatic system in the 21st century.

Besides, the RDA was never intended to advance health but only to prevent diseases like scurvy and rickets. It's done a great job with that. But taking the minimum amount of a nutrient to prevent gross-deficiency diseases doesn't help those people who want to be truly healthy and not just be free of symptoms. Optimal health should be the goal for all of us.

Most of our foods are processed, and therefore, the nutrients have been leeched out of them. Seventy percent of the population is deficient in magnesium, 65% are deficient in zinc, 48% are deficient in calcium, and 56% are deficient in Vitamin C. It's clear that everyone can benefit from taking a good multivitamin. The benefits have been reported in medical journals (literally thousands of studies), popular newspapers, and magazines. Taking a daily multivitamin and mineral formula reduces the incidence of heart disease, heart attack, stroke, glaucoma, macular degeneration, diabetes, senile dementia, and various cancers.

Many so-called experts will tell you not to worry about taking vitamins if you are eating a balanced diet: "Oh, you'll get all the proper nutrients you need." If you ever encounter a doctor who says this, simply smile and head for the nearest exit! By making such a statement, this physician has demonstrated that she is some twenty years behind in the research. How could someone who is supposed to be looking after our health be so ignorant to think that eating bleached bread, toxic meats, allergy-producing dairy products, and nutritionally void, simple carbohydrates could provide the necessary vitamins and minerals the body requires to be healthy? Remember, most medical doctors receive only three classroom hours of nutritional education!

However, their lack of classroom training shouldn't prevent them from staying abreast of latest findings that appear in their very own medical journals. Numerous studies published in the very journals these physicians are reading demonstrate the need for vitamin and mineral supplementation. It's no secret that our food supply is tainted with poisonous chemicals and laden with preservatives that rob the body of needed nutrients.

RDA Verses ODA

The chart on the following page shows a comparison of the two systems of recommendation as they apply to several common nutrients. (IU stands for international units.)

	RDA	ODA
Vitamin A	1,000 mcg.	10,000 mg.
Vitamin D	200 IU	100 IU
Vitamin E	15 IU	400 IU
Vitamin K	80 mcg.	60–80 mcg.
Vitamin B1	1.5 mg.	50–100 mg.
Vitamin B2	1.7 mg.	50 mg.
Vitamin B3	19 mg.	50 mg. (200 mg. if Niacinamide)
Vitamin B5	7 mg.	200–400 mg.
Vitamin B6	2 mg.	50–200 mg.
Folic Acid	200 mcg.	400–800 mcg.
Vitamin C	60 mg.	1,000–2, 0000 mg.
Calcium	800 mg.	500–1,200 mg.
Chloride	750 mg.	Not usually recommended
Chromium	50–200 mcg.	200–400 mcg.
Copper	1.5–3.0 mg.	1 mg.
Fluoride	1.5–4.0 mg.	Not usually recommended
Iodine	150 mcg.	Not usually recommended
Iron	10 mg.	Not supplemented unless anemic
Magnesium	350 mg.	500–1,000 mg.
Manganese	2.5–5 mg.	10–20 mg.
Molybdenum	75–250 mcg.	Same as RDA unless deficient
Phosphorus	800 mg.	Not usually recommended
Potassium	2,000 mg.	100 mg.
Selenium	70 mcg.	200 mcg.
Sodium	500 mg.	Not usually recommended
Zinc	15 mg.	25 mg.

More About Important Nutrients

Vitamin A is a potent antioxidant with immune-enhancing abilities. A deficiency in zinc ceases vitamin A metabolism, even when the vitamin is abundant. Too much vitamin A can lead to dry lips and skin, headache, thinning hair, and bone pain, but symptoms are quickly reversed when levels are reduced. White spots on the fingernails indicate a zinc and vitamin A deficiency and suggest reduced immunity. Especially important in FMS/CFS, vitamin A helps correct intestinal permeability (leaky gut). Leaky gut is associated with such allergic reactions as migraine, asthma, rheumatoid arthritis, irritable bowel, cystitis, sinusitis, rhinitis, ear infection, dermatitis, hives, and eczema. Vitamin A's other benefits include:

- developing and maintaining the surfaces of the mucous membranes, lungs, skin, stomach, and urinary, digestive, and reproductive tracts.
- maintaining a healthy thymus gland, which controls the entire immune system.
- helping to form bones and soft tissue, including tooth enamel.
- protecting against some cancers.
- treating acne (both orally and topically).
- enabling night vision.
- usefulness in calcium metabolism.
- protecting against asthma.
- reducing allergic reactions.
- helping prevent birth defects when taken by expectant mothers (a minimum of 2,000 IUs and no more than 8,000 IUs per day).

Beta-carotene can be converted into vitamin A, and beta-carotene is relatively nontoxic, whereas too much vitamin A can be quite dangerous. Beta-carotene is a group of caratenoids, which are found in dark green, yellow, and dark orange fruits and vegetables. It is a strong antioxidant with anticancer properties—one molecule of beta-carotene can destroy 1,000 free radicals. It protects the skin from harmful ultraviolet (UV) light. Women with low levels of beta-carotene in their cervical tissues are at risk for developing cervical cancer.

A 19-year study involving 3,000 men shows caratenoids (especially beta-carotene) may significantly reduce the incidence of lung cancer in both smokers and nonsmokers. (Studies have also demonstrated a 45% reduction in lung cancer in those individuals who take vitamin supplements.) Vitamin E and selenium enhance the role of beta-carotene. The only side effect of consuming too much beta-carotene is a yellowing of the skin, and this condition disappears once the intake is reduced.

Vitamin D is produced by the body after exposure to sunlight. It helps maintain healthy nerve and muscle systems by regulating the level of circulating calcium, which is essential for proper nerve transmission and muscle function. A deficiency in vitamin D can cause degeneration of bones and possibly hearing loss, if the small bones in the ear are involved.

Vitamin E is a major antioxidant that protects cells and tissues from oxidative stress. It also protects—from free-radical damage—the pituitary and adrenal hormones, fatty acids, and myelin sheaths surrounding nerves and genetic material. A deficiency in vitamin E can lead to heart disease, muscular dystrophy, nervous system disorders, anemia, liver damage, and birth defects. Smokers need to take extra vitamin E, since research at the University of California shows that vitamin E and vitamin C levels are reduced by exposure to cigarette smoke. Studies done in Israel show vitamin E can reduce the symptoms of osteoarthritis. Its other benefits include:

- preventing abnormal blood clotting.
- increasing the efficiency of muscles—including the heart—by reducing oxygen requirements.
- effectively reducing tension in the lower extremities, which is associated with intermittent claudication and heart disease.
- relieving restless leg syndrome or "the fidgets."
- helping to slow the aging process.
- increasing and maintaining proper brain function.
- helping protect the body from the toxic effects of lead and mercury.

Some evidence associates higher intake of vitamin E with a decreased incidence of cancer. The Iowa Women's Health Study has demonstrated a very strong protective effect for vitamin E. This was a large scale, four-year study of 35,000 women, age 55–66, who had no previous history of cancer. The results revealed convincingly that a high intake of vitamin E was associated with a reduced risk of colon cancer. Risk of colon cancer was reduced by 66% for women taking the highest amount of vitamin E.

The American Cancer Society recently released the results of a long-term study that evaluated the effect of vitamin E and C supplements on bladder-cancer mortality. The study followed 1,000,000 adults for a 15-year period and found that those who regularly consumed vitamin-E supplements for at least 10 years were 40% less likely to die from bladder cancer.

In one study, patients with moderately severe Alzheimer's disease were studied for two years. The patients were given either large doses (2,000 IU) of vitamin E, Eldepryl (selegiline hydrochloride), or a placebo for two years. In the patients who received vitamin E, there was a significant delay in disease progression. This study shows that Alzheimer's patients may live longer and remain in better health if they take high doses of vitamin E.

Vitamin E benefits those with type-2 diabetes, one of the most common diseases in the world. Researchers have found that oxidative damage may play a strong role in the damage to tissues caused by diabetes as well as in the complications of diabetes. The results show that when these patients took 400 IUs of vitamin E daily, they reduced their risk of heart attack by 43% and their risk of dying of heart disease by 55%. Since cardiovascular disease is the major cause of death in people with diabetes, vitamin E may have a strong, positive impact on health outcomes in diabetics.

Vitamin E lowers cancer risk in smokers. Scientists from the National Cancer Institute, working together with scientists in Finland, studied 30,000 male smokers in Finland. They found that of those who took a Vitamin E capsule every day for five to eight years, there was a 30% reduction in the cases of prostate cancer and a 40% reduction of deaths from prostate cancer. This is really exciting because in this country we expect about 40,000 men to die from prostate cancer this year.

During a four-year, double-blind study, not a single older person who took separate doses of vitamin E (200-800 IU) or vitamin C (500-1000 mg.) developed Alzheimer's disease. Subjects who took multivitamin supplements with low doses of vitamin E (typically 30 IU) or vitamin C (60 mg.) had no reduction in risk of Alzheimer's.

Taking 200 IU of natural vitamin E daily boosted immune functioning in older people. A supplement with only 60 mg. of vitamin E daily did not improve immune functioning. Obviously, superior immune functioning lessens infections, possibly cancer, and heart disease.

Many studies have uncovered the body's many uses of vitamin E.

Researchers at Tufts University found that on a diet supplemented with 200 IUs of vitamin E, control groups had a 65% increase in immune-fighting abilities. Researchers at Duke University have demonstrated that vitamin E acts as a potent antioxidant to counter the toxic effects of air pollution. (The amount needed to combat air pollution, including ozone and nitrous oxide, is six times the RDA.)

Selenium enhances the effects of vitamin E. A zinc deficiency increases the need for vitamin E. Vitamin E may be necessary for the synthesis of Vitamin B12. Vitamin E is relatively nontoxic, but taken in very high doses, it can cause interference with vitamin K and lead to prolonged bleeding. Vitamin E is safe, however, even when taken in dosages several times higher than the RDA. (The body stores fat-soluble vitamins, which include vitamins A, D, E, K, and beta-carotene. Because of this, an overdose is possible when taking these vitamins. However, the effects of vitamin toxicity are quickly eliminated once they are discontinued.)

Vitamin B1 (thiamin) is needed to metabolize carbohydrates, fats, and proteins. It is important for proper cell function, especially nerve cell function. It is involved in the production of acetylcholine, a nerve chemical directly related to memory and physical and mental energy. A deficiency of vitamin B1 can lead to fatigue, mental confusion, emaciation, depression, irritability, upset stomach, nausea, and tingling in the extremities. Vitamin B1 has been reported to be deficient in nearly 50% of the elderly. This could possibly explain the dramatic increase in presenile dementia and Alzheimer's disease the past few decades. Diets high in simple sugars, including alcohol, will increase the chances of a vitamin B1 deficiency. The tannins in tea inhibit vitamin B1 absorption.

Vitamin B2 (riboflavin) is responsible for the metabolism of carbohydrates, fats, and proteins. Vitamin B2 is involved in producing neurotransmitters, which are brain chemicals responsible for sleeping, mental and physical energy, happiness, and mental acuity. A deficiency of vitamin B2 can cause soreness and burning of the lips, mouth, and tongue; sensitivity to light; itching and burning eyes; and cracks in the corners of the mouth. Vitamin B2 can help curb the craving for sweets and is needed for the synthesis of vitamin B6. Vitamin B2 is needed to convert the amino acid tryptophan to Niacin (B3). Vitamin B2 is not absorbed very well, and any excess will turn the urine a bright fluorescent yellow. It is not toxic.

Vitamin B3 (niacin) plays an important role in mental health. Orthomolecular physicians have used niacin to treat schizophrenia, anxiety, and depression. It is a by-product of the metabolism of tryptophan. Some people have a genetic inability to breakdown or absorb tryptophan, and this can lead to aggressive behavior, restlessness, hyperactivity, and insomnia. Large daily doses of niacin can decrease LDL cholesterol and triglycerides while increasing the HDL.

Vitamin C (ascorbic acid) produces and maintains collagen, a protein that forms the foundation for connective tissue, the most abundant tissue in the body. Benefits of vitamin C include:

- fighting bacterial infections.
- helping wounds heal.
- preventing hemorrhaging.
- reducing allergy symptoms.
- helping to prevent heart disease.
- helping prevent free-radical damage.
- acting as a natural antihistamine.
- reducing blood pressure in mild hypertension.
- preventing the progression of cataracts.
- helping regulate blood sugar levels.
- possibly improving fertility.
- lowering LDL cholesterol while raising HDL cholesterol.
- increasing immune system function.
- helping the adrenal glands form important stress hormones.
- helping prevent toxicity of cadmium, a heavy metal that can increase the risk of heart disease.
- counteracting other heavy metals, including mercury and copper.

A deficiency in vitamin C can cause bleeding gums, loose teeth, dry and scaly skin, tender joints, muscle cramps, poor wound healing, lethargy, loss of appetite, depression, and swollen arms and legs. Vitamin C is important in the conversion of tryptophan to serotonin, and low serotonin levels are linked to insomnia and depression. A deficiency of vitamin C causes an increase in urinary excretion of vitamin B6 (also associated with making neurotransmitters). Aspirin, alcohol, antidepressants, anticoagulants, oral contraceptives, analgesics, and steroids can all interfere with vitamin C absorption. Ester C is absorbed four times faster than regular ascorbic acid. Most vitamin C is lost in the urine, but only one-third that amount of ester C is lost in urination. Pregnant women should not exceed 5,000 mg. in a day. Large doses of Vitamin C can cause diarrhea. I, along with many other nutritional experts, recommend gradually increasing vitamin C until you have a loose stool. Then, reduce your intake 500 mg. at a time until you no longer have diarrhea. This is your optimal dose.

Folic Acid is considered brain food. It is involved with energy production, synthesis of DNA, formation of red blood cells, metabolism of all amino acids, and production of the neurotransmitters, including serotonin. Folic acid needs vitamins B12, B3, and C to be converted into its active form. Low folic acid levels are associated with an increase in homocysteine, an amino acid linked to cardiovascular disease (vitamin B6, folic acid, and vitamin B12 all help reduce homocysteine levels). A deficiency in folic acid (one the most common vitamin deficiencies), will produce macrocytic anemia, digestive disorders, heart palpitations, weight loss, poor appetite, headache, irritability, depression, insomnia, and mood swings. A sore, red tongue may also indicate a folic acid deficiency. When taken by pregnant women, folic acid can improve an infant's birth weight, neurological development, and chances of escaping a neural tube defect. Women trying to get pregnant and expectant mothers should take a multivitamin with at least 400 mcg. of folic acid. Large doses of folic acid can mask a vitamin B12 deficiency.

Inositol is important in the metabolism of fats and cholesterol and in the proper function of the kidneys and liver. It is vital for hair growth and prevents hardening of the arteries. Inositol is needed for the synthesis of lecithin, which helps remove fats from the liver. Along with gamma-aminobutyric acid (GABA), inositol may help reduce anxiety. Caffeine may decrease inositol stores. There is no known deficiency or toxicity for inositol.

Para-aminobenzoic acid (PABA) is needed to form red and white blood cells, which in turn, form essential B vitamins. PABA is used in suntan lotion to help block harmful UV rays and prevent sunburn. PABA has antiviral properties and has been reported to help in treating Rocky Mountain spotted fever. PABA may help restore gray hair to its natural color. PABA and sulfa drugs cancel each other out. Doses over 1,000 mg. can cause nausea and vomiting.

Boron is needed in trace amounts for the proper absorption of calcium. A recent study by the US Department of Agriculture showed women who consumed 3 mg. of boron a day lost 40% less calcium and one-third less magnesium in their urine. Excessive amounts of boron can cause nausea, diarrhea, skin rashes, and fatigue.

Calcium is the most abundant mineral in the body. It comprises 2–3 pounds of total body weight and is essential for the formation of bones and teeth. Calcium regulates heart rhythm, cellular metabolism, muscle coordination, blood clotting, and nerve transmission. Adequate intake of calcium can help lower high blood pressure and the incidence of heart disease. Calcium contributes to the release of neurotransmitters. It can also have a calming effect on the nervous system. A deficiency of calcium can result in hypertension, insomnia, osteoporosis, tetany (muscle spasm), and periodontal disease.

The ratio of calcium-to-magnesium and calcium-to-phosphorous is important. Recommended ratios are 2 to 1 (or 1.5 to 1) for calcium to magnesium and 2 to 1 (or 3 to 1) for calcium to phosphorous.

Vitamin D is needed for the absorption of calcium. Calcium absorption is decreased by high protein, fat, and phosphorous (junk food) diets. Chelated calcium (bound to a protein for easier absorption) and magnesium can help reduce aluminum and lead poisoning. Excessive calcium intake (several grams a day) can cause calcium deposits in the soft tissue, including the blood vessels (causing arteriosclerosis) and kidneys (causing stones). Oyster shell or bone meal calcium supplements often contain high levels of toxic lead. Calcium citrate or ascorbate are recommended instead.

Chromium is involved in the metabolism of blood sugar (glucose). It is essential in the synthesis of cholesterol, fats, and protein. Chromium helps stabilize blood sugar and insulin levels. Proper interaction between blood sugar and insulin insures proper protein production, reducing the chance for fat storage. A deficiency in chromium can cause type-2 diabetes, hypoglycemia, and coronary artery disease. Ninety percent of the US population is deficient in chromium! Diets high in simple sugars increase the loss of chromium, and a deficiency can cause a craving for sugar. Zinc can inhibit chromium absorption and should always be taken separately. Chromium is not toxic.

Copper maintains the myelin sheath, which wraps around nerves and facilitates nerve communication. It plays a vital role in regulating the neurotransmitters and helps maintain the cardiovascular and skeletal systems as well. It is part of the antioxidant enzyme supraoxide dismutase and may help protect cells from free-radical damage. Copper helps with the absorption of iron, and a deficiency in copper can lead to anemia, gray hair, heart disease, poor concentration, numbness and tingling in the extremities, decreased immunity, and possibly scoliosis.

Cadmium, molybdenum, and sulfate can interfere with copper absorption. A niacin deficiency can cause an elevation of copper. Zinc and copper impair the absorption of one another, so they should be taken separately. Intake of 20 mg. or more in a day can cause nausea and vomiting. Wilson's disease is a genetic disorder characterized by excessive accumulation of copper in the tissues, as well as liver disease, mental retardation, tremors, and loss of coordination.

Iron is important in formation of hemoglobin, oxygen use, energy production, muscle function, thyroid function, and components of the immune system, protein synthesis, normal growth, and mental acuity. Excessive amounts of vitamin E and zinc interfere with iron absorption. Vitamin C helps with the absorption of iron. Vitamin B6 is needed to develop the iron-containing protein hemoglobin. Iron should not be routinely supplemented; a blood test should first confirm an iron deficiency. The exception would be females who rigorously exercise. Studies show that only 8% of the US population is deficient in iron. However, 20% of premenopausal women and as much as 80% of women who exercise are deficient in iron. People suffering from Candida and chronic herpes infection usually have a deficiency in iron. If you suspect you have an iron deficiency, ask your health professional for a blood test. Excessive amounts of iron are associated with an increased risk of heart disease and can lead to decreased immunity and liver, kidney, and lung disorders.

Magnesium is one of the most important minerals in the body. It is responsible for proper enzyme activity and transmission of muscle and nerve impulses, and it aids in maintaining a proper pH balance. It helps metabolize carbohydrates, proteins, and fats into energy. Magnesium helps synthesize the genetic material in cells and helps to remove toxic substances, such as aluminum and ammonia, from the body. Adequate amounts of magnesium are needed to ensure proper heart function. Magnesium and calcium help keep the heart beating; magnesium relaxes the heart, and calcium activates it. A deficiency of magnesium may increase the risk of heart disease. Magnesium also plays a significant role in regulating the neurotransmitters. A deficiency in magnesium can cause depression, muscle cramps, high blood pressure, heart disease and arrhythmia, constipation, insomnia, hair loss, confusion, personality disorders, swollen gums, and loss of appetite. High intake of calcium may reduce magnesium absorption. Simple sugars and/or stress can deplete the body of magnesium.

Magnesium is a natural sedative and can be used to treat muscle spasm, anxiety, depression, insomnia, and constipation. It is also a potent antidepressant. It helps with intermittent claudicating, a condition caused by a restriction of blood flow to the legs. Magnesium is also effective in relieving some of the symptoms associated with PMS, and women suffering from PMS are usually deficient in magnesium—as is 80% of the general population. New studies are validating what many nutrition-oriented physicians have known for years: a magnesium deficiency can trigger migraine headaches.

Magnesium helps relax constricted bronchial tubes associated with asthma. In fact, a combination of vitamin B6 and magnesium, along with avoidance of wheat and dairy products, has cured many of my young asthmatic patients. Normal dosage is 500–800 mg. daily. Too much magnesium can cause loose bowel movements. If this occurs, reduce your dose.

Manganese aids in the development of mother's milk and is important for normal bone and tissue growth. It is involved in the production of cellular energy, metabolizes fats and proteins, and is essential in maintaining a healthy nervous system. Manganese is needed to synthesize thiamin, and it works in coordination with the other B vitamins to reduce the effects of stress. A deficiency of manganese can cause fatigue, impaired fertility, retarded growth, birth defects, seizures, and bone malformations. Calcium, copper, iron, manganese, and zinc all compete for absorption in the small intestine, and large doses of one of these nutrients may reduce the absorption of the others. Many of my patients who suffer from CFS/FMS are deficient in manganese. It is not toxic. Recommended dosage is 5–15 mg. daily.

Molybdenum aids in the conversion of purines to uric acid and allows the body to use nitrogen. It is important in sulfite detoxification and promotes normal cell function. Molybdenum deficiency can cause stunted growth, loss of appetite, and impotence in older males. Excessive copper may interfere with molybdenum absorption. Molybdenum works with vitamin B2 in the conversion of food to energy. Molybdenum can help reduce symptoms associated with sulfite sensitivities. I had a patient who broke out in a rash every time she ate foods containing the preservative sulfite. A hair analysis revealed a molybdenum deficiency. Once her molybdenum levels were normalized, she was once again tolerant of sulfites. High dosages can cause symptoms similar to gout: joint pain and swelling. Recommended dosage is 50–150 mcg. daily.

Potassium, sodium, and chloride help to regulate the nervous system and heart rhythm. These three minerals are known as electrolytes due to their electrical charge. They are responsible for maintaining a proper pH (along with calcium and magnesium). Excess sodium can cause an elevation in blood pressure. Potassium helps lower blood pressure and can reduce the risk of stroke. Chloride helps make up the digestive enzyme hydrochloric acid. Hydrochloric acid helps digest food, destroys harmful intestinal "bugs," and synthesizes vitamin B12. Chronic diarrhea, vomiting, heat stroke, prolonged use of diuretics, and kidney disease can cause a deficiency of all three of these minerals. A potassium deficiency manifests itself as irregular heart beats, sterility, muscle weakness, apathy, paralysis, and confusion. A chloride deficiency can lead to alkalosis, an imbalance in the body's pH system. This imbalance can cause vomiting and more diarrhea. A sodium deficiency is rare, but it can occur after long periods of sweating, fasting, and/or diarrhea. Sodium increases urinary calcium loss, while potassium decreases urinary calcium loss. Potassium and magnesium are synergetic in lowering blood pressure and, therefore, should be taken together.

Selenium is an important antioxidant that protects the body from free-radical damage. It is a component of glutathione peroxidase, an enzyme essential for detoxification of cellular debris. Selenium, along with other antioxidants, especially vitamin E, combats free radicals that can cause heart disease. Selenium may help prevent certain forms of cancer and help those suffering from autoimmune disorders such as rheumatoid arthritis. It is an important component of the immune system. It helps make thyroid hormones and essential fatty acids. A deficiency can cause birth defects, certain cancers, and fibrocystic, heart, and liver disease. Doses above 600 mg. can cause side effects that include tooth decay and periodontal disease. Recommended dosage is up to 200 mcg. daily.

Zinc is important in over 90 enzymatic pathways. Zinc facilitates alcohol detoxification within the liver. It plays a role in producing and digesting proteins. Zinc is also important in maintaining normal blood levels of vitamin A, boosting the immune system, healing wounds, converting calories to energy, reducing low birth rates and infant mortality, controlling blood cholesterol levels, and producing the prostaglandin hormones that regulate heart rate, blood pressure, inflammation, and other processes. A deficiency of zinc can lead to poor taste, anorexia nervosa, anemia, slow growth, birth defects, impaired nerve function, sterility, glucose intolerance, mental disorders, dermatitis, hair loss, and atherosclerosis. Excess copper can cause a zinc deficiency, and vice versa. Pregnant women accumulate excess copper and become zinc-deficient. This can lead to postpartum depression. Extra zinc, 50 mg. per day, should be consumed by pregnant females to help avoid unwanted postpartum depression. Zinc lozenges have been shown to reduce the symptoms and duration of colds by 50%. It is estimated that 68% of the population is deficient in zinc. Zinc deficiency can cause depression, since it's necessary for the production of dopamine. Fingernails that contain white specks are indicative of a zinc deficiency. Recommended dosage is up to 50 mg. daily.

Index